Praise f
A Dignified

"*A Dignified Life* is a compassionate, well-written and extremely valuable resource. Using the Best Friends approach outlined in the book, caregivers are provided with a wide range of practical tools and strategies for how to deal with the many challenges of coping with this difficult disease. I highly recommend *A Dignified Life* both for professionals and family caregivers."

—Ken Dychtwald, PhD
CEO and founder of Age Wave

"Alzheimer's disease causes anguish to millions of caregivers and family members. Few diseases are feared more, with its loss of memory, identity and ability to recognize loved ones. It is these loved ones who must face enormous responsibilities that they are seldom prepared to handle alone. *A Dignified Life* is supportive and practical, offering a down-to-earth, comprehensive approach for providing care for people with Alzheimer's."

—Robert N. Butler, MD
founding director of the National Institute on Aging and Pulitzer Prize–winning author of *Why Survive? Being Old in America*

"The Best Friends approach was a miracle for our family. My mother thrived on this friendship approach at her day center, and this affirming philosophy helped me through some difficult times. I can definitely recommend this book to anyone on the journey of dementia. I've become a big advocate for Best Friends."

—Jan Cerel
Caregiver (Lexington, KY)

"As a gerontologist, I hear from families every day about the challenges of Alzheimer's care. Virginia and David's Best Friends approach is full of helpful advice, success stories, tips, and techniques for turning failure into success. It's the best book on Alzheimer's care!"

—Amy S. D'Aprix, MSW, PhD, CSA
founder of Essential Conversations, Inc., and author of
From Surviving to Thriving—Transforming Your Caregiving Journey

"This life affirming and positive philosophy brings dignity to our residents with dementia, our staff, and our families at Prestige Care. A wonderful book full of wisdom and success stories."

—Hollie Fowler
Senior Director Product and Brand Development, Prestige Care

"Helping patients and families cope with Alzheimer's disease is one of the major challenges for our society. Bell and Troxel have provided an outstanding guide for anyone involved in the care of individuals with Alzheimer's disease. The Best Friends method is an innovative, sensitive, and unique approach that can greatly improve the quality of life for patients with the most devastating disease known to humankind."

—William R. Markesbery, MD
past director, Alzheimer's Disease Research Center and
Sanders-Brown Center on Aging, University of Kentucky

"We know that people with dementia and their caregivers have some of the same essential needs regardless of country, culture, or traditions, and we know that using a person's life story is the key to meeting those needs. The Best Friends approach to dementia care beautifully articulates this universal truth and supports Home Instead's 'to us it's personal' philosophy. It is highly recommended!"

—**Jeff Huber**
president and chief operating officer, Home Instead Senior Care

"Truly a must read for all those who care for people with dementia. *A Dignified Life* is packed with effective and practical advice and full of humanity. It shows that there is much that can be done to help make the lives of both caregivers and people with dementia better and more fulfilling. I give it a five-star rating."

—**David Snowdon, PhD**
author of *Aging with Grace*

"As a neurologist, I dream about the day that we will find a cure for Alzheimer's disease. Until that time, the Best Friends approach is here to give families practical tools for bringing out the best in persons with Alzheimer's disease. This is a well-written, insightful book that gives caregivers a life-affirming, practical framework for approaching this difficult disease. I recommend it to my patients and their families."

—**Donna Masterman, MD**
medical director, Genentech, Inc.

"Caregivers can easily become overwhelmed by the daily challenges facing them. The Best Friends approach will give you simple, easy-to-learn tools that can make the most daunting problems seem easier to cope with. I highly recommend this book."

—**Elaine St. James**
author of the international book series *Simplify Your Life*

"T. S. Eliot once described friendship as 'the inexpressible comfort of feeling safe with a person having neither to weigh thoughts nor measure words.' Virginia Bell and David Troxel succeed in describing the many aspects of friendship necessary for helping a loved one to journey safely through Alzheimer's disease when ordinary thoughts and words often fail. Families will find this to be a useful guide."

—Daniel Kuhn, MSW
author of *Alzheimer's Early Stages* and *The Art of Dementia Care*

"Virginia Bell and David Troxel are leaders in the field of aging. Their words will offer caregivers new ideas and new hope as they face the challenge of Alzheimer's disease and dementia."

—Gloria H. Cavanaugh
former president and CEO, American Society on Aging

"For every friend, relative, or caregiver to a person with Alzheimer's, *A Dignified Life* offers practical advice, compassion, and optimism in understanding and dealing with the challenges they face each day and on how to bring out the best in the person with the disease, so that a life that seems at times hopeless can be a life of love and dignity."

—Jack Canfield
author of *Chicken Soup for the Unsinkable Soul*

"The Best Friends book is my 'go to' resource for helping families and professionals caring for persons with dementia. Virginia Bell and David Troxel have created a life affirming and easy to use philosophy of care that brings out the best in the person with dementia. The Best Friends approach can turn around behaviors that are challenging, support good communication, and help care partners create a successful day."

—Elizabeth Edgerly, PhD, chief program officer,
The Alzheimer's Association, Northern California
and Northern Nevada Chapter

A DIGNIFIED LIFE

REVISED AND EXPANDED

A DIGNIFIED LIFE

REVISED AND EXPANDED

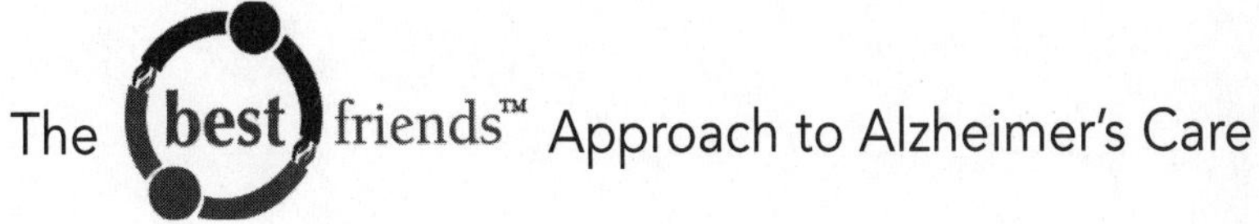

The best friends™ Approach to Alzheimer's Care

A GUIDE FOR CARE PARTNERS

Virginia Bell and David Troxel

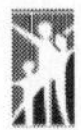

Health Communications, Inc.
Deerfield Beach, Florida

www.hcibooks.com

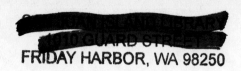

Library of Congress Cataloging-in-Publication Data

Bell, Virginia.
A dignified life, revised and expanded : the best friends approach to Alzheimer's care : a guide for care partners / Virginia Bell and David Troxel.—Rev. and expanded.
p. cm.
ISBN 978-0-7573-1665-4 (pbk.)
ISBN 0-7573-1665-4 (tradepaper)
ISBN 978-0-7573-1666-1 (e-book)
1. Alzheimer's disease—Patients—Long-term care. I. Troxel, David. II. Title.
RC523.B434 2012
616.8'31—dc23

2012033306

A Dignified Life: The Best Friends Approach to Alzheimer's Care, Revised and Expanded is a trade original, based on the authors' earlier work, The Best Friends Approach to Alzheimer's Care (©1997, 2003, 2012 in press by Health Professions Press, Inc.).

This Health Communications, Inc., edition is published by arrangement with Health Professions Press, Inc., Post Office Box 10624, Baltimore, Maryland, 21285-0624, USA. Information on other books on The Best Friends approach may be found at www.healthpropress.com/bestfriends.

Publisher: Health Communications, Inc.
3201 S.W. 15th Street
Deerfield Beach, FL 33442-8190

Cover design by Erin Geoghegan
Interior design and formatting by Lawna Patterson Oldfield

To the many persons with Alzheimer's disease or other dementia who have inspired us with their courage, and to their care partners, who have inspired us with their commitment, wisdom, and loving care.

To our friends and colleagues around the world who work every day to help families, while dreaming of a world without Alzheimer's.

CONTENTS

II THE BEST FRIENDS APPROACH

III THE BEST FRIENDS APPROACH IN ACTION

ACKNOWLEDGMENTS

We have many people to thank who have stood by us since we first began our work in Alzheimer's disease and dementia care in the mid-1980s.

Our friends and colleagues at the Sanders-Brown Center on Aging at the University of Kentucky deserve special acknowledgment. Dr. David Wekstein first brought us together as colleagues, and the center and its talented staff grew under the leadership of its late director Dr. William R. Markesbery. Other Sanders-Brown staff and alumni to thank include Dr. Deborah Danner, Robin Hamon, Dr. Linda Kuder, and Marie Smart.

Tonya Cox of Christian Care Communities has been a longtime friend and collaborator.

We thank the staff and volunteers at the Best Friends Day Center (Lexington, Kentucky) for their ongoing commitment to this outstanding model program. This award-winning adult day center was the birthplace of the Best Friends approach and remains an influential source of learning and inspiration.

Two chapters of the Alzheimer's Association have provided a home and support for us in our work. The Greater Kentucky and Southern Indiana Chapter of the Alzheimer's Association was an early pioneer in adult day center care, notably the development of the national model program Helping Hand (now the Best Friends

Center), and we thank all of the volunteers and talented staff who have worked with us in Kentucky, notably Claire Macfarlane, Marie Masters, Jane Owen, Margaret Patterson, and Ray Rector. The California Central Coast Chapter of the Alzheimer's Association encouraged and supported the work of David Troxel, and we thank this organization's past and present committed staff and volunteers, notably Charlie Zimmer, Barbara Rose, Lol Sorensen, Elayne Brill, Dr. Erno Daniel, Dr. Robert Harbaugh, and Julian Dean.

Other notable supporters include Dr. Linda Hewitt, who provided guidance on sexuality and dementia, and Joanne Rader, who shared expertise on issues surrounding bathing. The Robert Wood Johnson Foundation first funded us in our adult day center care work in Lexington, Kentucky; without its support, much of our work on Best Friends would not have occurred. Dr. William Stivelman of the Mary Oakley Foundation has supported our ideas with grants that have allowed our work to be translated into Spanish and for outreach into the Latino community. We also appreciate the support of the many friends we have met through Alzheimer's Disease International, notably Dr. Nori Graham and Dr. Lilia Mendoza.

Our earnest appreciation goes to Anne Basye of Mount Vernon, Washington, who has ably facilitated Best Friends' leap into social media by supporting and creating a website and Facebook page.

Finally we thank the team at HCI—Allison Janse, Kelly Maragni, Lori Golden, and Kim Weiss—for all their efforts in producing this revised edition. Special thanks to the team at Health Professions Press—Melissa Behm, Mary Magnus, and Julie Chávez—for their support and friendship.

—The Authors

To the many Best Friends Day Center volunteers in Lexington, Kentucky, who have exemplified the Best Friends approach since 1984, and to my husband, Wayne Bell, and our children, grandchildren, and great-grandchildren, who have had to live with a nontraditional wife, mother, grandmother, and great-grandmother in order for this book to be published.

—Virginia Bell

I thank my many old and new friends working in the field of dementia care and the families I have met who are traveling the Alzheimer's journey. I also thank my partner, Ronald Spingarn, and my late parents, Fred and Dorothy Troxel, who cheered me on with unconditional love and support.

—David Troxel

INTRODUCTION

Receiving a diagnosis of Alzheimer's disease or other dementia is devastating news, both for the person being diagnosed and for his or her friends and family. Dementia gradually robs individuals of their memory, judgment, language, and eventually their physical health. It takes away a person's independence. Dementia also can prove devastating for husbands, wives, partners, adult children, and other family members. Caring for a person with dementia may mean giving up your career, balancing the needs of your own children with dementia care, or postponing dreams of "the golden years" of retirement to face the often physically and emotionally stressful task of providing supervision, support, and care.

Yet, there is reason for optimism. A worldwide research effort is under way to conquer Alzheimer's disease and other dementia. More support groups, educational programs, day centers, and specialized residential and in-home support programs are being developed all the time. We are also learning so much about how to interact with the person with dementia. Contrary to what many people believe, much can be done to improve the lives of people with Alzheimer's disease to help them feel safe, secure, and valued—to help them live a life with dignity—and, in turn, create a more meaningful and manageable experience for caregivers.

When this book was first published in 2002, it represented the first comprehensive approach or philosophy of care written just for families. The book had a simple premise—that what a person with dementia needs is a best friend, someone who understands, is supportive, communicates, and encourages activity and engagement. The Best Friends™ approach and this book enjoy continued popularity because the philosophy it presents is easy to learn, understand, and apply to your caregiving experience. This approach has helped thousands before you and will help you recast or rethink your own life supporting a friend or family member with dementia, transforming caregiving from a burden to a more rewarding and successful experience with fewer frustrations. Learning the Best Friends approach will teach you what we call "the knack" of providing good care; the art of doing difficult things with ease.

The Best Friends approach will give you valuable insights and skills for your caregiving journey. Irene Elam, who embraced the Best Friends approach in her husband's care, sums up her experience in this way: "From early on, I made up my mind to do three things: I wasn't going to raise my voice, I wasn't going to argue, and I was going to keep my sense of humor any way I could." You can begin to travel the same journey that Irene traveled. Let's take a look at the Best Friends approach:

- *Understanding what it's like to have dementia*: Behaviors that seem strange or unreasonable become quite understandable when you know their origins. The Best Friends approach suggests that having empathy and knowing what is causing a behavior allows you to give individuals with dementia what they need when they need it, whether it's reassurance, physical contact, or something that helps them "save face."

- *Knowing and using the person's life story*: Persons with Alzheimer's disease forget much of their past. It is important for us to be their biographers and know and use the life story. This helps us recall happy times and successes (Dad's hole in one on the golf course) and also redirect the person when he or she is having a bad day (calming agitation by asking Mom to teach you how to make her famous apple pie).
- *Knowing just what to say when communication is breaking down*: Alzheimer's disease damages the ability of a person to understand and be understood. When the person with dementia is in his or her home of thirty years saying, "I want to go home," or is telling you that she has just had a bath when she has not bathed in a week, the Best Friends approach offers practical tips, examples, and guidelines that can help. There is a wrong way and right way to communicate with a person with dementia.
- *Offering the right activities in the right way*: Because persons with dementia may no longer be able to take part in activities they once enjoyed, or initiate new ones, they can easily become isolated, bored, and frustrated. The Best Friends approach will help you understand the importance and purpose of activities and offer ideas to stay engaged throughout the day.
- *Supporting a spiritual or religious life*: As dementia progresses, it can become difficult for the person to stay connected to a past spiritual life. The Best Friends approach honors the spiritual life of all persons. You will find many ways to nurture the spirit through art, music, and nature, in addition to religious

faith. Spiritual traditions, rituals, and activities can continue throughout the illness.

- *Being your own Best Friend*: Many individuals giving care become so consumed with their roles that their own physical and emotional health suffer. They stop doing the things they once enjoyed and become as isolated as the person in their care. The Best Friends approach will help you develop a personal strategy for maintaining your own well-being, even while facing one of the most difficult challenges life can dish up.

* * *

The Best Friends approach was first described in a book originally published in the late 1990s, *The Best Friends Approach to Alzheimer's Care* (Health Professions Press, 1996), written for professionals working in long-term care settings. Much to our surprise, however, the first comment we received after the book was published was not from a nursing home administrator or a day center director, but from a woman with early-stage Alzheimer's disease. Ruth McReynolds told us that our book had helped her become more accepting and optimistic about her future. Since that time, we've met many persons like Ruth who have expressed their appreciation for the inherent dignity of the Best Friends approach.

An early advocate for our approach was Elayne Brill, founder of the Alzheimer's Association in the greater San Francisco Bay Area, who claims to have "lived through the dark ages of Alzheimer's." When she cared for her husband George in the 1980s there was almost no public information or support. "I wasn't prepared to be open to a more positive approach to this terrible disease, but I embraced

Virginia and David's Best Friends philosophy. It all began to make sense. I never thought I'd say it, but you can come out on top."

We knew that the Best Friends approach wasn't just for professional caregivers, but for family caregivers like Elayne as well. *A Dignified Life* was written to speak more directly to the circumstances and needs of families that are thrust into a caregiving role by this disease.

The stories of the transformative effects of the Best Friends approach are boundless. Rita West Paustian's is just one example.

> *I struggled when my mom was diagnosed, as I live in Auburn, Washington, and felt increasingly guilty because I wasn't there to help my Dad [in Kansas]. Also, I realized I was "losing" my mother. On one of those visits, my Dad gave me information about Best Friends, which quickly became my "bible." I had often wondered how Dad seemed to know just how to engage my mother so that she continued to feel needed and loved. . . . He was putting your ideas into practice. My mother's life, as well as ours, was enriched during that difficult time thanks to everything we learned about being a Best Friend.*

Putting the Best Friends approach into practice helped Rita's father be a more empathetic and successful husband, and it helped Rita make the most of her visits with her mother.

Best Friends has been embraced in formal care settings and by professionals around the world. Programs in Australia, Brazil, Canada, Finland, Germany, Great Britain, Hungary, Italy, Lebanon, South Africa, and Taiwan are among many other countries using our approach to care. The books have been translated from English into seven languages. In the United States, a number of state governments now consider the Best Friends approach a "best practice" and are providing Best Friends training to long-term care providers and families. Alzheimer's Association chapters and groups ranging from Maine to Oregon have embraced the philosophy of care, offering conferences, workshops, online programs, and training curricula. Long-term care providers including residential care companies and in-home providers have also adopted the philosophy. EMTs and paramedics have received Best Friends training; it helps them make a connection and provide reassurance and comfort even in times of crisis. Dr. Nori Graham, a physician and past chair of the London-based organization Alzheimer's Disease International, sums up quality dementia care in a way that is very much in keeping with the spirit of the Best Friends approach: For Dr. Graham, the key to successful dementia care is "informed love," and success comes from knowledge mixed with a caring, gentle attitude and approach.

This revised edition of *A Dignified Life: The Best Friends Approach to Alzheimer's Care* contains insights from individuals who are using the Best Friends approach every day. It also reflects new ideas and trends in dementia care. The new edition:

- Reflects upon contemporary ideas and trends that have emerged since its original publication in 2002. We now know so much more about the "other dementias" (for example, vascular dementia, frontotemporal dementia, Lewy body and Parkinson's-related dementia, and others). This book expands its discussion of these dementias.
- Offers more tips and suggestions on how to manage behaviors that are challenging.

- Expands upon the benefits of engagement and activity—both planned and spontaneous. We now know that activities including exercise and music along with lifelong learning are good for all of us, including persons with dementia.
- Offers new stories from many of the persons with dementia and their families we have met during the past ten years, including some professionals who have embraced this philosophy of care in their own work.
- Explains new resources and services for families, including the rise in hospice care as a key service for persons with dementia.
- Describes surprising ways to use the Internet for activities and engagement.
- Introduces the Best Friends website (www.bestfriendsapproach.com), which can update you on our work and provide a forum for our readers to share their own success stories and questions.
- Updates suggested online and community resources.

A Dignified Life is written to help you rethink your approach to care, learn how to be a Best Friend to the person you are concerned about, and approach your role with more confidence, skill, and success. By applying what you learn from reading this book, we hope that you and your loved one will soon discover that, truly, a Best Friend can provide the best care.

The book draws from a wealth of experience working directly with people with dementia and their friends and families, including our work with local chapters of the national Alzheimer's Association, a university research center, dozens of in-home and residential and day center care providers, and the Best Friends Day Center program in Lexington, Kentucky. The Best Friends Day Center, opened in 1984 under the name The Helping Hand Day Center, was one of the first dementia-specific adult day programs created in the country and has become a model program, in large part because it embodies the Best Friends philosophy. Many of the examples in this book are drawn from our experiences with the center's participants and their families.

There are a number of important ways in which this book differs from other books you can find on Alzheimer's care.

First, the authors have adopted a positive, optimistic outlook. We share many success stories that will help you learn how to avoid falling into the trap of hopelessness and helplessness. In dementia care there are typically good days and bad days. The Best Friends approach will help you have more good days.

Second, all stories mentioned in this book are real and include the full names of the people involved. We do this to reduce the stigma of Alzheimer's disease, to bring it out of the darkness. We worried that families would be uncomfortable telling their stories, but when we asked them for written permission they all agreed. They did this to remember or honor their loved ones and to support a greater understanding of dementia. We commend them for their openness and encourage the reader to learn more about the real people we feature by reading their short "Biographies" at the end of the book.

We would like to draw the reader's attention to the following points:

- While much of the public focus has been on Alzheimer's disease, this book looks at "Alzheimer's disease *and other dementia*" and we use that language throughout. The word *dementia* is an umbrella term encompassing many diseases and disorders that impact thinking, language, memory, and brain health. The Best Friends approach applies to any dementia.

- We introduce a term that may be new for readers of this book who are familiar with the commonly used word *caregiver*. In this book we choose to use the phrase *care partner* to describe those friends and family members who are there for the person with dementia. This term is in wide use internationally and is making its way into the United States. It reflects a contemporary view that the person with dementia still has much to offer if given the opportunity and in the right way; they *can* be a "partner" in their own care. We understand that it may not always be an *equal* partnership—caregivers often have to do most of the chores, driving, cooking, helping the person in the shower, and much more—but the Best Friends approach will help you build cooperation so that care is less one-way.
- All authors writing in this field struggle with describing the man or woman with dementia. In this book, we use *person(s)* to describe individual(s) with Alzheimer's disease or other dementia. We hope this will be more economical to the reader than other phrasing. At the same time, this term gently reminds us that there is a person beneath the cloak of dementia, one who has feelings, one who has led a life full of rich experiences, and one who deserves a dignified life.

As we have revised this edition, one disappointment has loomed large. While basic research has advanced, no breakthrough drugs have emerged. The brain is proving an amazing, but complex organ.

Solving its mysteries and finding truly effective ways to prevent, treat, or cure Alzheimer's disease and other dementia still elude us.

Until we can create a world without dementia, the Best Friends approach continues to work its magic in homes and programs around the world. We hope that it also supports you and your journey.

Virginia Bell, MSW
David Troxel, MPH
August 1, 2012

I

ALZHEIMER'S DISEASE AND OTHER DEMENTIA

1

WHAT'S HAPPENING?

The Experience of Alzheimer's Disease and Other Dementia

What is it like to have Alzheimer's disease and other dementia? What would it be like to be unsure of your surroundings, to have difficulty communicating, to not recognize a once-familiar face, or to be unable to do things you have always enjoyed? When you understand the world of people with dementia, you can begin to understand their experiences, develop empathy, and relate better to their situations.

The experience of Alzheimer's disease and other dementia can be like taking a trip to a foreign country where you don't speak the language. Customs are different. Deciphering a restaurant menu proves difficult; you may think you are ordering soup and end up with fish! When paying a restaurant bill with unfamiliar currency you might fear that you are being shortchanged, cheated. Tasks so easy at home are major challenges in an unfamiliar setting and can be exhausting. The person with dementia is in a foreign land all the time, as seen in Irene Hong's postcard.

6-30-95 RECEIVED JUL 10 1995

Hello Friends!
Rural Taiwan is lush & green, but I'm staying in the noisy city of Taipei in my grandmother's place, who's 80 & sharp as a nail. One thing that might interest you is that when my Mom 1st came back to Taiwan after a 20 yr-ascence, she was so disoriented that she surmised this might be what the initial stages of A.D. is like. She couldn't find the right words in Taiwanese (her native language) & she'd forgotten some of the customs, though everybody expected her to know her way around her "home" country. She felt so frustrated! It is true that A.D. is like travelling in a foreign country, isn't it?
Irene Hong

Alzheimer's Association
Virginia Bell
801 S. Limestone St., Suite E
Lexington, KY 40508
U.S.A.
PAR AVION

TAIWAN

Hello Friends:

Rural Taiwan is lush and green but I'm staying in the noisy city of Taipei in my grandmother's place who is 80 and sharp as a nail. One thing that might interest you is that when my Mom first came back to Taiwan after a 20 year absence, she was so disoriented that she surmised this might be what the initial stages of Alzheimer's is like. She couldn't find the right words in Taiwanese (her native language) and she'd forgotten some of the customs though everybody expected her to know her way around her "home" country. She felt so frustrated. It is true that Alzheimer's disease is like traveling in a foreign country, isn't it?

Irene Hong, volunteer,
Postcard sent to Helping Hand Day Center

Rebecca Riley was one of our early teachers about the experience of dementia. A nurse and educator, Rebecca was diagnosed with Alzheimer's disease at age 59. When she first began having difficulty teaching, she thought it was because the course content was new. Soon, she knew something was wrong with her thinking and memory, and she suspected that she might have Alzheimer's disease. Her physician later confirmed her suspicions. Rebecca taught us about the world of dementia. Following are some of her written notes describing her experience:

- Depression
- Can't say what I want
- Afraid I can't express my thoughts and words—thus I remain silent and become depressed
- I need conversation to be slowly
- It is difficult to follow conversation with so much noise
- I feel that people turn me off because I cannot express myself
- I dislike social workers, nurses, and friends who do not treat me as a real person
- It is difficult to live one day at a time

Rebecca knew that she was losing her language skills and the ability to communicate her wishes. Her writing reveals that her once-meticulous grammar was slipping. Complexity became her enemy; she could not follow the din and roar of competing conversations—calling it "noise." Her statement about social workers, nurses, and friends who do not treat her as a "real person" still makes us both smile and wince. Even though her cognitive skills were in decline, she recognized that people were treating her differently. Consequently, she expressed her anger and some resentment toward these people. Remarkably, she was trying to create a plan for the future. Her notes indicate that she was deciding to take things "one day at a time" even if it was a struggle.

Reading these heartfelt words, you too can begin to understand the experience of Alzheimer's disease and other dementia. Without understanding this world, we cannot possibly develop successful strategies for improving the lives of our friends or loved ones with dementia.

Emotions That Accompany Alzheimer's Disease

Persons with dementia commonly experience these emotions and feelings:

- Worry and anxiety
- Frustration
- Confusion
- Loss
- Sadness
- Embarrassment
- Paranoia
- Fear
- Anger
- Isolation and loneliness

COMMON EMOTIONS AND FEELINGS OF PERSONS WITH ALZHEIMER'S DISEASE AND OTHER DEMENTIA

Every person's response to Alzheimer's disease or other dementia is different, but many people will experience one or more of the following emotions.

Worry and Anxiety

We all worry or become anxious at times. Parents worry and become anxious about their teenager who is not home by curfew. Families may worry about having enough money to pay all of their bills at the end of the month. Some people worry that a favorite celebrity's marriage is in trouble after reading the latest tabloid at the supermarket.

The person with dementia can become consumed by worry and anxiety. One frequent by-product of dementia is that the person cannot separate a small worry from an all-consuming concern. For example, a person with dementia may begin worrying about dark clouds in the sky seen through a window. Left unchecked, the worry can grow and wreck his or her afternoon. A spring shower could turn into a thunderstorm!

Harry Nelson was a practicing dentist when he was diagnosed with Alzheimer's disease in his mid-fifties. He was very anxious about his life and the lives of his family. He worried, when in spite of his determination to keep fit mentally, spiritually, and physically, his scores on his mental exam kept going down. He worried that he would not be able to go hiking with his grandson when he became old enough to enjoy a sport that he loved. His dreams and aspirations were on hold, and he had difficulty not being anxious about the future.

Harry's worries are typical of many people with dementia. They may become upset if they think they're not meeting their employment obligations or are late for work. This makes sense: work consumes much of our lives, and it's understandable that this part of a person's life will still resurface on occasion.

Frustration

Almost all of us occasionally misplace car keys. The keys turn up eventually, but the search can be very frustrating. Imagine the frustration of losing your keys or wallet every day, every hour.

Because short-term memory is attacked, the person with dementia may constantly be looking for something he or she is certain has been misplaced. Frustration may also stem from failing to complete everyday tasks. In the morning, a thoughtful care partner may leave clothes on the bed for her mother with Alzheimer's disease. Her mother stares at the underwear, blouse, a skirt, a sweater, shoes, and jewelry. What goes on first? What may have once been so simple is now an elaborate series of steps performed in a certain sequence: put on the hose before the shoes, the bra before the blouse. Yet, because she loses her ability to sequence, this woman with dementia finds that the simple act of dressing is extremely frustrating. On top of this, the person is easily tired out or exhausted by the extra effort and concentration it takes to complete a once routine task.

Accustomed to using his reasoning and problem-solving abilities in his work, Brevard Crihfield or "Crihf," the former executive director of the Council of State Governments, summed up his experience of Alzheimer's disease when he said in frustration, "It is like my head is a big knob turned to off."

Crihf's description of Alzheimer's disease remains one of the best we've heard; it is powerful and articulate.

Confusion

What do you think when a friend does not show up for a lunch date? Maybe one of you got the time and date mixed up. You hope nothing serious has happened, so you try calling your friend's cell phone, and the mystery is solved—you have gone to different restaurants! The confusion has been cleared up, but if your friend had not answered his telephone, you would still be at the restaurant, waiting impatiently.

For many people with dementia, confusion is a daily experience. The person is never quite sure about anything—the time of day, the place, and the people around him or her. Also, unlike the above example, people with dementia often cannot sort out or work their way through the confused state.

Ruby Mae and a volunteer at a day center were looking at a photo album. "Look, Ruby Mae, you are dancing with a handsome young man." Ruby Mae loved a good time and seemed to be enjoying reliving some fun times. When it was time to eat, she insisted that they bring "him" to lunch, too. "Him?" the friend wondered. "You know that nice one we were just dancing with. He's hungry too," Ruby Mae replied.

Ruby Mae was profoundly confused, but she kept her sense of humor throughout her long journey with Alzheimer's disease.

Loss

Many of us define ourselves by our jobs, our relationships, or the things we do. You might say, "I am proud to be a good carpenter," "I am Wayne's mother/father," or "I am a fly fisherman." If any of us had to make a major change in life and these roles were taken from us, we would experience feelings of great loss.

People with dementia lose these titles and, as a result, lose important and meaningful roles. Eventually, they will be unable to work and will have to give up favorite activities. Sooner or later, the losses mount.

Sometimes, as care partners, we tend to focus on our own losses (e.g., the relationship, the time consumed by caregiving, the hard work that can accompany physical care) and forget to acknowledge the losses of the person. But it is important to remember that the person with dementia experiences painful loss day after day.

Learning to Understand

A simple exercise can help you begin to understand the impact of dementia. Take five small pieces of paper. On each piece, write one of your favorite activities. A typical activity might be visiting the grandchildren, taking a day trip in the car, enjoying a favorite hobby, going to work, trying a new recipe, playing golf, or talking on the phone with an old friend. After you are through, select an activity, think about how much you enjoy it, and then imagine giving it up. Take the piece of paper listing the activity, wad it up, and throw it away. Continue to do this until you have discarded all five pieces. How do you feel?

The odds are that you are now experiencing the feelings of loss that many with dementia feel. Sadly their losses are real, not "paper losses." Worse, they cannot choose the things to give up. That choice has been made by Alzheimer's disease or other dementia.

Dr. John "Jack" Cooper had a distinguished career as a Navy commander and surgeon. He would say, "I don't have a job. I don't have any money. I don't have my life anymore."

In spite of Jack's many losses, he still remembered being and was very proud to be a physician. He preferred to be called "Jack" day-to-day, but liked to be introduced as "Dr. Cooper" on special occasions.

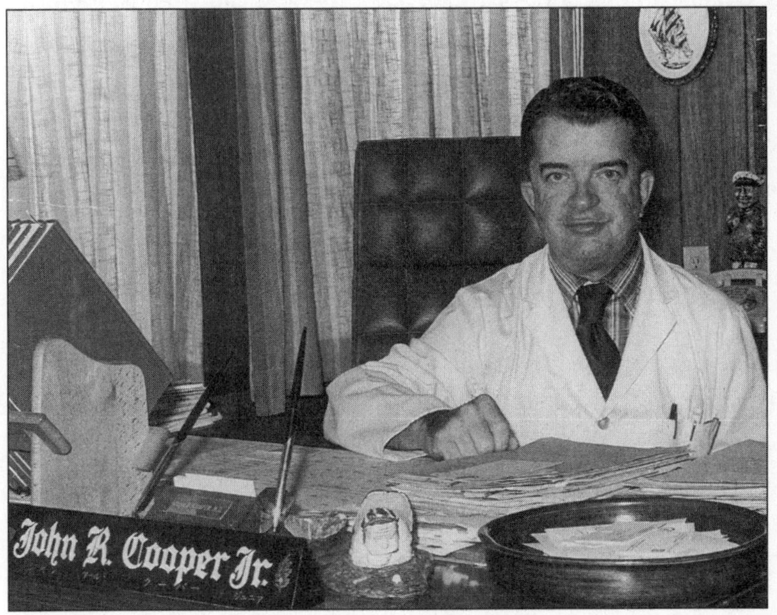

Dr. John Cooper at the height of his medical career, 1971

Sadness

All of us experience moments of sadness. Perhaps you remember a failed relationship or the loss of a beloved pet. Maybe a poignant story on the news makes you teary. Sadness can be fleeting, or it can be long-lasting and associated with a profound grief process. Like happiness, sadness is a part of life.

Feelings of sadness are often pervasive among people with dementia. A person can burst into tears at the thought of not being able to tell a story all the way through or at forgetting a name. A person can also feel sad over long-term losses, such as having to move out of a family home. People who do not have dementia can develop strategies to overcome sadness (seek therapy, call friends, go for a hike); people with dementia lose this ability to work their way out of sadness.

Geri Greenway was at the peak of her career as a college professor when she was diagnosed with Alzheimer's disease in her late forties. Aware of the nature of the disease, she often sat with her hands covering her eyes, as if her world was too painful to see.

Being diagnosed so young created intense feelings of sadness for Geri, but she responded enthusiastically to smiles, hugs, and friendly, reassuring words.

Embarrassment

All of us can remember a time in school when the teacher called on us and we did not know the answer to a question. You might recall your collar tightening, voice faltering, palms sweating, and face blushing.

The person with dementia is in a giant classroom every day, one in which he or she never has the exact answer. A woman who always prided herself on her appearance may have someone point out that she is wearing her jacket inside out. Names are easily forgotten.

Embarrassment is common for persons with dementia, particularly those who are more aware of their mistakes.

"There she is! When did she come in? That's my wife over there." Hobert Elam was sure that he had spotted his wife at the day center at a table across the room. When he approached her, he realized it was not his wife and was very embarrassed. "I can't believe that I made that mistake," he admitted to a volunteer at the program.

Mixing up identities is a common occurrence for people with dementia. They begin to forget faces and sometimes can be confused when people look alike. They may confuse genders, thinking a woman with short hair is a man and that a man with long hair is a woman. Declining vision and hearing can make the situation worse. When the person knows he or she has made a mistake, it can be embarrassing.

Paranoia

If your boss starts treating you differently, you may wonder if he or she is unhappy with your performance. If you see a strange car outside your house several days in a row or if someone is standing too close to you at the ATM as you're withdrawing money, you may become alarmed. Even the most well-grounded individual becomes a bit paranoid in some circumstances.

People with dementia often look for an explanation about what is happening to them. Why does their family refuse to let them drive? Where is their money? When they cannot find rational explanations, they sometimes experience bouts of paranoia, imagining that someone is trying to harm or hurt them in some way. Delusions or fixed, false ideas are extremely common in persons with the most common dementia, Alzheimer's disease. Paranoia can be a by-product of these delusions.

Emma Simpson kept complaining to her daughter, Patricia, that the woman next door was taking her scissors. Emma was sure of it because she could never find a pair of scissors when she needed them. One day, Patricia moved her mother's purse and it was heavier than she could imagine. She began unloading the purse and found seventeen pairs of scissors of every kind, color, and description, making the purse bulge at the seams.

Hoarding or hiding things is common for persons with dementia. They may be paranoid that someone is stealing things or simply be trying to keep track of their valued possessions, like Emma.

Fear

All of us become fearful now and then. Perhaps you're walking in a big city late at night and hear footsteps behind you. Maybe you're afraid of earthquakes or tornadoes, spiders or snakes.

Individuals with dementia also have fears. These may include the loss of independence, placing too much burden on family members, and getting lost. Other fears might include traumas from the past that have risen again in the present (e.g., thinking that a Vietnam War event is still happening) and fears caused by delusions (someone is stealing their money). Misperceptions of vision or space can subsequently lead to a fear of falling, particularly if the carpeting on the floor has a confusing or misleading pattern.

Sisters Henrietta and Mae Frazier lived together for many years. Henrietta's cheerful disposition made it easier for her sister to care for her—except that after her diagnosis of Alzheimer's disease Henrietta developed a terrible fear of bathing. Whether it was the running water, the cold porcelain tub, or some past trauma, she was often reduced to tears when being helped with her bath.

Mae was able to address this fear by hiring a particularly sensitive home health aide, who took plenty of time and built a trusting relationship with Henrietta. (See page 190 for some ideas about bathing.)

Anger

All of us get angry occasionally, and although no one wants to bear the brunt of it, anger has a constructive purpose: It can help us fight a battle if threatened. It can release harmful stress and pent-up emotion. Also, sometimes getting something off your chest by becoming angry can lead to healing in relationships.

It is a myth that all, or even most, people with Alzheimer's disease are violent. Yet people with dementia can become angry. They may not always understand what is happening around them and to them. Anger can also stem from a loss of control when they feel rushed or unduly pressured to do something.

"You go home!" Annie yells if angered. Her husband, Jack Holman, says that she has always been very independent, and that now, having to depend on others for all her needs is really difficult for her. Because of her Alzheimer's disease, her vocabulary is very limited, but she still can find words to express herself when she becomes angry.

Persons like Annie may continue to have angry moments, but learning to use the Best Friends approach can help care partners understand the triggers for her anger and learn ways to cope.

Isolation and Loneliness

A friend of the authors hurt his leg in a skiing accident and had to curtail most of his activities for a month. He could not go to the office, could not work out at the gym, had to give up his opera tickets, and had to cancel outings with friends. He told us that he was very lonely during his recuperation. His first day back at work was one of the happiest of his life.

As Alzheimer's disease progresses, isolation and loneliness often increase. The person can no longer drive and may no longer be able to play a weekly bridge game, go sailing with friends, do woodworking, go shopping, or even walk down to the neighborhood doughnut shop. The person loses social contacts; worse yet, friends eventually stop visiting. Unlike a broken leg, the person's memory cannot be mended.

> *A former teacher and community leader, Rubena Dean often felt left out of activities. She once said, "I used to play cards, I used to drive, I used to work . . . there are too many 'used tos' in my life now."*

Despite not knowing who the president of the United States was, what day it was, or even how old she was, Rubena was surprisingly articulate about what it is like to have dementia.

Early-Stage Support Groups

More and more organizations are now offering support groups not just for caregivers but also for individuals with dementia. These groups range from social, "club-like" meetings to ones that include more therapeutic elements. The individual with dementia responds to the camaraderie, the humor, the sharing, and the feeling that he or she is not alone. Even families who thought that their loved ones would never try such a group have been impressed. Another variation on these groups is what some groups call a "Memory Café." Learn about that program on page 228.

With dementia, friends tend to fall away. When a person with dementia meets another person going through the same experience, an instant friendship often forms and feelings can be shared and discussed.

Several books and newsletters are available that discuss these groups and are listed under Organizations, Websites, and Recommended Readings (page 283).

THE BEST FRIENDS APPROACH

Now that you've read this chapter, take a moment to imagine what it is like to have dementia. Try doing the simple Learning to Understand exercise (page 20)—it is a powerful tool for care partners and can help you better understand the person's frustration and anger.

You are a lucky care partner if you do not bear the brunt of these feelings from time to time. Fortunately, many people with dementia also feel happy and joyful at times. These feelings can be momentary or long-lasting. Sometimes the very losses of dementia provide a level of emotional protection that insulates them from the problems of the world, their family, or even their disease. Thus, the person with dementia can have moments throughout the day when he or she is enjoying the company of a pet, savoring a piece of chocolate, laughing at a joke, or celebrating a mutual hug. Sometimes with humor and sometimes with guilt, care partners have admitted in support groups that their loved one's personality has changed for the better. The overachieving, aggressive, "type-A" father sometimes becomes more playful; the pessimistic aunt becomes an optimist; the uptight, controlling mother learns to relax.

CONCLUSION

This book outlines the Best Friends approach to caring for a loved one with Alzheimer's disease and other dementia. The Best Friends approach can help you understand the feelings expressed by people with dementia. As the saying goes, to understand someone, you must "walk a mile in his shoes." When you walk this mile—or run this marathon, as many care partners feel—you begin to see one of the underlying surprises of this book: The so-called inappropriate behaviors of dementia are not all that mysterious or out of place. They often stem from the person's efforts to make sense of his or her world, to navigate the maze of dementia. If any of us experienced memory or judgment problems, if any of us were afraid of something, if any of us had to give up most or all of our favorite activities, it would be perfectly normal to be sad or anxious, to hide things, to wander away from a possibly threatening situation, to leave the house if we think we're late for work, or to strike out at someone we think is trying to hurt us.

Once you understand what underlies the challenging behaviors, you begin to see dementia care in a new light. The Best Friends approach helps you gain this perspective. And remember: because the person's medical condition will not change, it is we, as friends and family, who must change.

Best Friends Pointers

- Feelings of loss, confusion, frustration, and anger can be normal feelings caused by dementia.
- People with dementia are working very hard to make sense of their world, to see through this confusion and memory loss.
- Taking time to think about the experience of the person helps us overcome denial, develop empathy, and be a more supportive and effective care partner.

2

WHAT IS KNOWN?

Diagnosis, Treatment, and Research

Learning the basics about the medical and scientific aspects of Alzheimer's disease and other dementia is an important part of being an effective care partner; it helps you understand that dementia is real and gives you the tools needed to implement the best plan of care. You do not need to become an expert on dementia research, but staying well informed will help you provide care more confidently. In addition, by better understanding the disease's impact on the person, you learn to separate the person from his or her disease and to focus your feelings—your anger and frustration, for example—on the disease instead of on the person.

This chapter contains key concepts about memory loss, Alzheimer's disease, and other dementia, including information about diagnosis, treatment, and research, all of which will help you better understand the condition experienced by your loved one. As we get older, almost all of us are concerned about our own memory and cognitive well-being, so the information in this chapter is also for anyone concerned about his or her own situation.

Because research is progressing so rapidly, there will be ongoing and important developments after the date of publication of this book. Organizations, Websites, and Recommended Readings, on page 283, includes contact information for various newsletters, nonprofit groups, and useful websites to help you stay up to date.

Ten Warning Signs of Alzheimer's Disease

1. Memory loss that disrupts daily life
2. Challenges in planning or in solving problems
3. Difficulty completing familiar tasks
4. Confusion with time and place
5. Problems with visual images and spatial relationships
6. New problems with words in speaking or writing
7. Misplacing things and losing the ability to retrace steps
8. Decreased or poor judgment
9. Withdrawal from work and social activities
10. Changes in mood and personality

From *Ten Warning Signs of Alzheimer's Disease*, © 2009, National Alzheimer's Association. Used with permission.

IS IT NORMAL TO HAVE MEMORY LAPSES NOW AND THEN?

Everyone forgets names now and then or forgets why they've just walked into a room. One way to determine if you have a memory problem is through the following tongue twister:

If you remember forgetting, that's okay.
If you forget you forgot, that's not.

An individual who forgets to buy several items he or she needs at the grocery story generally does not have a problem. If he or she makes an implausible excuse for the mistake ("The grocery store was out of milk and bananas" or "Someone stole them from my shopping cart"), there is reason to be concerned.

Forgetfulness is not the only sign of a potential problem. Sometimes apathy, personality changes, or the inability to learn and use new information can mark the beginnings of a dementing illness. See the ten warning signs of Alzheimer's disease on page 32.

CAN A DOCTOR HELP SOMEONE DETERMINE IF THERE IS A PROBLEM?

Whatever someone's age, if there are signs of memory loss, confusion, or other cognitive problems, a medical examination is recommended. Consulting a doctor early if you have a problem or concern is essential not only because treatments early in the Alzheimer's disease process may help postpone later stages, but also because you may have a reversible disorder.

Today, most physicians are up to date on dementia and are capable of conducting a basic evaluation; however, many families prefer to be referred to a neurologist or a geriatrician for a specialist's opinion. Either way, an evaluation should include a thorough medical history, a neurological examination, a neuropsychological or mental status exam, a brain scan, lab tests, and any other tests the doctor deems necessary. Testing may include a computerized tomography (CT) or magnetic resonance imaging (MRI) scan to look for signs of problems in the brain such as stroke, normal pressure hydrocephalus, or tumors. Some workups include a positive emission tomography (PET) scan that can record the brain functioning in "real time" and offer a dramatic look at areas of the brain not "lighting up" as they should.

Some people with early signs of dementia cover up symptoms. They often retain social skills and manners and can fool everyone around them, at least for a while. A sensitive medical practitioner can see through this. For example, a neuropsychological exam commonly asks the patient to recall words, name items commonly found in a kitchen, count backward by sevens, draw pictures of a clock face, and recall other information that is hard to "cover up." Families sometimes are shocked by the results that clearly show that the person's cognition has deteriorated more than they thought; perhaps the mother who was a homemaker and wonderful cook is socially appropriate but can only name three things in a kitchen during the test—for example, a toaster, refrigerator, and stove.

WHAT DOES IT MEAN IF THE DOCTOR DIAGNOSES SOME FORM OF DEMENTIA? IS THAT THE SAME AS SENILITY?

Senility is an out-of-date word that basically just means "old." It is not used today in the medical profession because it reinforces many stereotypes about aging, particularly the notion that everyone who gets old "loses his or her mind." The preferred term now is *dementia*, originating from the Latin word meaning "away from mind." Dementia is the universally accepted term to describe losses in intellectual functioning including one or more of the following: memory loss, language deficits, diminished judgment, declining problem solving, and lack of initiative. Many people detest this term, saying that it is a depressing word, or sounds like craziness. We don't particularly

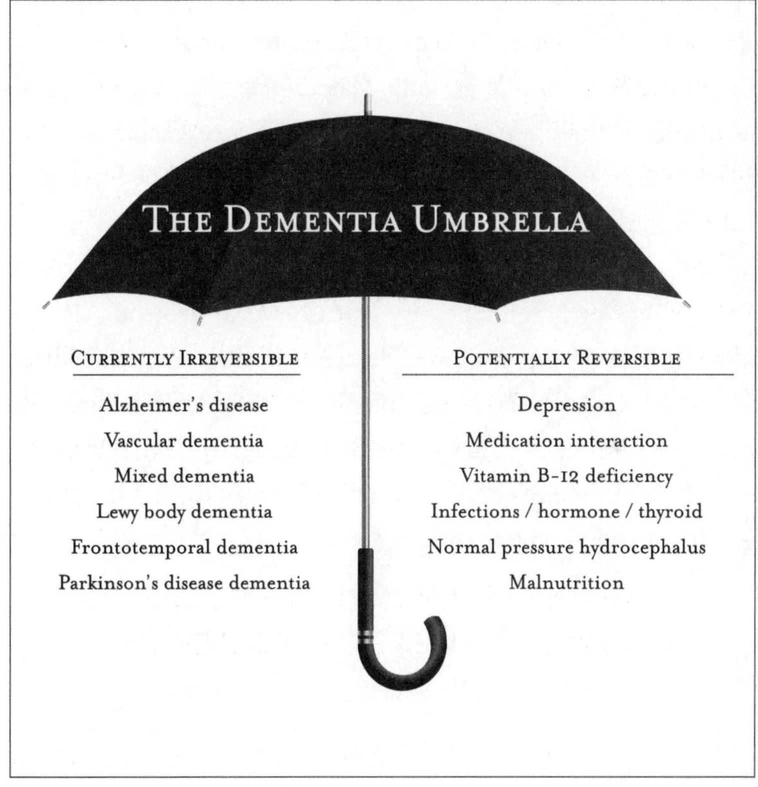

Illustration courtesy of Matthew Ehrmann.

like it either, but for now it is the most accepted word that medical professionals use.

By itself, dementia is not a complete or an appropriate diagnosis; dementia is a syndrome. Someone who sees a doctor should expect to have a diagnosis that describes a specific type of dementia and should be assured that treatable or other causes of cognitive loss have been excluded. Each form of dementia has a slightly different appearance and course. To help explain this concept, imagine the word "dementia" on a large umbrella. Underneath that umbrella, the disorders that can cause reversible and irreversible dementias are listed. As you can see on the previous page (The Dementia Umbrella), Alzheimer's disease is just one form of dementia.

Another way of explaining the word "dementia" is described by Carol Bowlby Sifton. She says that the word "dementia" is like the word "soup." Soup is a broad description; there are many kinds of soup, such as tomato, mushroom, or chicken noodle. Similarly, dementia is a broad description and there are many kinds of dementia, such as Alzheimer's disease, vascular, Lewy body, and the others we will learn about in this chapter.

DISORDERS THAT MAY BE REVERSIBLE

The following disorders may be treatable, or even reversible.

- **Depression**: This is a condition marked by sadness, inactivity, difficulty with thinking and concentration, feelings of hopelessness, and, in some cases, suicidal tendencies. Depression can often be reversed with medical treatment and counseling.
- **Medication interactions**: Many older individuals take a variety of prescription and over-the-counter medications. Misuse of these, or use of medications that are not compatible, can cause symptoms of dementia.
- **Infections**: Left unchecked, infections such as urinary tract infections or even an infected tooth can cause symptoms of dementia. Fortunately, these problems usually respond to medical attention.
- **Vitamin B_{12} deficiency:** Low levels of this vitamin and folic acid can cause symptoms of dementia. Treatment can often improve or reverse the dementia.
- **Hormonal disorders**: Very low or very high levels of thyroid hormone can cause symptoms of dementia. Correcting the problem will usually reverse these symptoms.
- **Normal pressure hydrocephalus (NPH):** This is a rare disease caused by an obstruction in the flow of spinal fluid. Symptoms include difficulty in walking, memory loss, and incontinence. NPH is often correctable with surgery.
- **Malnutrition:** When someone does not eat well, he or she can actually become malnourished. This is particularly a problem when a frail elderly individual lives alone. At its worst, malnourishment can contribute to dementia.

DISORDERS THAT ARE CURRENTLY IRREVERSIBLE

Alzheimer's disease (discussed in detail starting on page 39) is by far the most common irreversible dementing illness; however, other dementias are receiving more and more attention as we now know that they are more common than once realized.

- **Vascular dementia** results from brain damage caused by the interruption of blood flow to the brain or multiple strokes (infarcts) within the brain. Symptoms can include disorientation, confusion, and behavioral changes. Vascular dementia is neither reversible nor curable, but treatment of underlying conditions (e.g., high blood pressure) may halt progression.
- **Mixed dementia** is a common diagnosis that involves the person having both Alzheimer's disease and vascular dementia.
- **Lewy body dementia:** Usually, Alzheimer's-like symptoms are present in the beginning of this disease, along with abnormal movements associated with Parkinson's. Other symptoms include hallucinations and delusions, falls, and bouts of unconsciousness (almost like a "swoon"). Individuals with Lewy body disease can also be very sensitive to psychotropic medications. Cholinesterase inhibitors may help (see page 43).
- **Frontotemporal dementia**: This dementia affects the frontal lobes of the brain. Pick's disease is one such disorder. Symptoms include (sometimes extreme) personality and behavioral changes that may precede memory loss. Interestingly, the peak age for this dementia is 55 to 65, and it is the only dementia that affects more men than women. Modern imaging techniques are helping detect these dementias.

- **Parkinson's disease dementia:** This disease affects control of motor activity, resulting in tremors, stiffness, and speech impediment. About 20 percent of people with Parkinson's develop dementia, usually after ten to fifteen years of living with Parkinson's. Parkinson's drugs can improve motor control but don't treat the cognitive losses.
- **Creutzfeldt-Jakob disease (CJD):** A rare, fatal brain disease caused by infection; a variant of this is the infamous "mad cow" disease. Symptoms include failing memory, changes in behavior, and lack of muscular coordination. CJD progresses rapidly, usually causing death within one or two years. No treatment is currently available.
- **Huntington's disease:** This hereditary disorder is characterized by irregular movements of the limbs and facial muscles, a decline in thinking ability, and personality changes. It can be positively diagnosed, and symptoms can be controlled with drugs, but the progressive nature of the disease cannot be stopped.
- **Korsakoff's syndrome:** In most cases, individuals with Korsakoff's syndrome have been abusers of alcohol. In its most severe form, the affected individual can only recall items from long-term memory and has no ability to form new memories.

THE MOST COMMON DEMENTIA—ALZHEIMER'S DISEASE

Alzheimer's disease was described initially in the early 1900s by a German doctor, Alois Alzheimer (1864–1915), for whom it was named. Now a famous case in the history of medicine, his patient

Auguste Deter began having symptoms of dementia at age fifty-one. Her symptoms included irrational jealousy toward her husband, trouble with cooking and handling money, paranoia, and anxiety. Auguste died four years later after progressive deterioration. When Dr. Alzheimer, a neuropathologist, did a brain autopsy, he found evidence of the neurofibrillary tangles and plaques that mark the disease as we now know it. The case became widely known when a colleague of Dr. Alzheimer published it in a handbook of psychiatry in 1910; from that point on, it was known as "Alzheimer's disease."

Alzheimer's disease has probably always been present but has become widespread more recently with increased longevity and the resulting aging of the U.S. population (and other countries). Although younger people are affected, the disease primarily affects individuals sixty-five years of age and older. Most experts say that approximately 15 percent of people over sixty-five will develop Alzheimer's disease or other dementia and 40 percent of people over eighty-five. Younger people do get dementia; an estimated 500,000 have Alzheimer's disease or other dementia under the age of 65.

According to the National Alzheimer's Association, "Alzheimer's disease usually begins gradually, causing a person to forget recent events and to have difficulty performing familiar tasks. How rapidly the disease advances varies from person to person, causing confusion, personality and behavior change, and impaired judgment. Communication becomes difficult as the person with Alzheimer's disease struggles to find words, finish thoughts, or follow directions. The hallmark of Alzheimer's disease is memory loss—notably short-term memory—followed by other cognitive deficits." Over time, individuals with Alzheimer's disease generally become unable to care for themselves, which creates enormous demands on family and professional care partners.

There currently is no definitive test for Alzheimer's disease, although work in this area is advancing rapidly. Some doctors will give a diagnosis of "probable Alzheimer's disease" if someone is showing a slow, progressive decline in cognition and if tests have ruled out other causes. More and more, however, doctors are dropping the word "probable," believing that a thorough evaluation can almost always be relied upon.

Do All People with Alzheimer's Disease Have the Same Course of Illness?

There can be tremendous variations in how Alzheimer's disease affects a person. Some individuals progress rapidly, others slowly. Some have almost all the classic hallmarks of dementia, including diminished visual/spatial perception, judgment, language skills, and short- and long-term memory; others retain more strengths and skills for long periods of time.

If You Have Alzheimer's Disease or Other Dementia

If you have received a diagnosis of Alzheimer's disease or other dementia it is important to get help from a reputable organization that can help you navigate the journey. See Organizations, Websites, and Recommended Readings on page 283 for a number of recommendations. Support groups or social groups for persons with dementia are highly recommended and increasingly common. You may be interested in a growing network of persons with early-stage dementia, called

Dementia Advocacy and Support Network International (DASNI), on the Web at www.dasninternational.org. Many of these individuals are assuming the role of activists to get more services and support. They also provide a support system for each other through personal contacts, telephone calls, and the Internet.

In addition, be sure to ask your physician about trying any of the memory-enhancing medications on the market, try to stay physically and intellectually active, get your legal and financial affairs in order, execute a durable power of attorney for health care, create a living will, and stay optimistic about future new treatments.

Even in the same person, the symptoms and behaviors change over time. This is a good news/bad news situation for care partners: The good news is that problems that seem daunting sometimes diminish or end; for example, paranoia, aggression, or wandering may diminish or go away over time. The bad news is that care would be easier if the future could be predicted. The typical length of illness is eight years from when the disease's symptoms begin to impact daily life to the time of death; although this, too, can vary widely.

Many clinicians speak about three "stages" of Alzheimer's disease. In Stage 1, or early stage dementia, the person may still be able to perform everyday tasks but is gradually having a decline in memory, problem solving, language, and judgment. In Stage 2, or the middle stage, the person's symptoms become much worse, and he or she needs ongoing supervision and support. Also at this point, the person begins to have trouble managing daily life, becomes lost in a familiar neighborhood, stops paying bills, leaves the stove on, or becomes a victim of financial abuse due to diminished judgment.

In the final or late stage, Stage 3, the person develops physical manifestations such as major incontinence, problems in swallowing, and other physical difficulties.

These stages are somewhat arbitrary but can be a useful clinical tool. We recommend that families not focus on a particular stage but instead recognize that Alzheimer's is typically slow and progressive, that people have good and bad days, and that every person has differing strengths and weaknesses.

What Kind of Medical Treatment Is Appropriate?

Memory-enhancing medications that may help persons think more clearly and perform daily activities more easily are on the market and recommended for people in early and middle stages of Alzheimer's disease and other dementia. Some physicians are now calling Alzheimer's disease and many of the related dementias treatable, but not reversible. The most common medications (Aricept, Exelon, and Razadyne) function as cholinesterase inhibitors; these drugs improve symptoms of the disease by helping to boost the brain's neurotransmitters—chemicals essential to thinking and memory that are depleted in Alzheimer's disease. Another drug, Namenda, works differently but seems to also help; most of the time it is used in combination with a cholinesterase inhibitor.

Studies suggest that drugs are most effective when started early in the disease process. These drugs may also positively affect behavior and do not add to the person's confusion, as do many psychotropic drugs (discussed on page 45). Encouragingly, new classes of drugs will continue to go on the market that will attack Alzheimer's disease and other dementia in other ways. It is important to remember, however, that these drugs do not offer a cure. Still, every person diagnosed with dementia should be evaluated to see if these memory-enhancing medications would be helpful.

Can Other Health Problems Worsen the Effects of Dementia?

Yes. Some medical or health-related conditions will, if left untreated, increase a person's dementia (these are called "medical excess disabilities"). An example is the person whose treatable vision problem has not been addressed, thus increasing disorientation and confusion. Getting this person new glasses would eliminate this excess disability. Other examples of treatable problems include urinary tract infections, constipation, pain (perhaps from a headache or a toothache), dehydration, and depression (which often accompany Alzheimer's disease).

Recognize that sudden changes in mood, energy, or behavior can be indicative of physical problems unrelated to the dementia. If a woman with Alzheimer's disease who is usually alert and happy suddenly becomes angry and acts out, it is possible that she is in pain and cannot name it; she may not be able to say that she has a toothache or stomachache. She might even have a more serious medical problem needing immediate attention. Thoughtful care partners recognize that a "behavioral" problem might be a medical condition that, once treated, will allow the person to function at his or her full potential. See Health Problems That Play Havoc, page 45.

What Are Psychotropic Drugs and Can They Help?

Psychotropic drugs are mood-altering drugs. They can make an enormous difference when extreme behaviors occur (sleeplessness, intense anxiety, dangerous paranoia, frightening delusions). Psychotropic medications can also drastically improve a care partner's ability to keep a loved one at home or help a person stay in assisted living and interact with other residents more positively. Because of the potential for serious side effects, they should be used judiciously and only after environmental or behavioral approaches have failed. For example, one family discovered that increasing the lighting in mother's house reduced her paranoia; psychotropics were not necessary.

However, finding the right medication and right dosage for older, frail individuals with dementia is challenging. To use an old nursing expression, "start low and go slow" if you are using psychotropic medications.

Health Problems That Play Havoc

Many health problems can increase or exaggerate the symptoms of dementia and should be treated if detected:

- Infection
- Medication issues or errors
- Depression
- Pain
- Hearing loss
- Heart problems
- Uncontrolled diabetes
- Dehydration
- Nutritional problems
- Vision loss
- Toothaches/mouth problems
- Food problems
- High/low blood pressure
- Hypothermia
- Bowel/bladder problems

Some drugs that effectively treat anxiety, hallucinations, delusions, sleeplessness, or aggression may increase confusion or overly sedate the person; many also have other unacceptable side effects, including added fall risk.

It's important to first try behavioral approaches to managing dementia (as described throughout this book) whenever possible. Being a Best Friend and offering creative activities along with "hugs instead of drugs" can often address these behaviors without the need for psychotropic medication. If you are using these medications, some doctors recommend periodic "medication holidays" to determine if the problem for which it was originally prescribed has been resolved.

Is Alzheimer's Disease Inherited?

Alzheimer's disease does run in some families (thus, it can be called a *familial* disease), but a person's children, siblings, or other relatives may never develop it (thus, it is not considered an inherited disease). The consensus among researchers is that an individual's chances of developing Alzheimer's disease are somewhat higher if a parent had the disease, particularly if the parent's onset came at a younger age (e.g., forties through sixties). Yet, even if someone is at genetic risk for developing it, the disease might not ever manifest itself. There is also optimism that the enormous strides being made in research will lead to preventive methods, a treatment, or even a cure.

Mild Cognitive Impairment (MCI)

Many doctors are using a new term—mild cognitive impairment (MCI)—to describe subtle memory loss seen in older individuals. An example of a person with MCI might be someone who handles personal care unassisted, walks to a favorite restaurant without getting lost, orders off the menu with confidence, and easily calculates a 15 percent tip when paying the bill, yet who asks the same question three times during dinner. The person is doing well cognitively except for a major deficit in memory.

For some, a diagnosis of MCI might be Alzheimer's disease at its earliest stage. For others, it might be "benign memory loss" and not worsen significantly over time.

Intense research continues and there is some hope that we may soon discover ways that individuals with MCI can be helped by interventions that will improve memory and/or prevent losses from progressing further.

Can Alzheimer's Disease Be Prevented?

There is currently no known way to prevent Alzheimer's disease, although researchers see this as an area of great hope. It is likely that Alzheimer's disease may actually develop years before symptoms appear; early detection might improve the chances of developing effective early interventions. Our hope is that a medical or lifestyle intervention will be discovered that will delay or prevent the onset of Alzheimer's disease.

Aspects of lifestyle that are modifiable and seem to offer hope include exercise, diet, and social engagement. Some studies have suggested that people who exercise regularly may get Alzheimer's disease later in life than those who do not exercise. Another possible preventive factor is diet; eat your antioxidant-rich green leafy vegetables and fruit. The Mediterranean diet that is rich in seafood, olive oil, and vegetables (with less red meat and dairy) may be helpful. Social engagement is also a factor. People who have friends and stay socially engaged may get Alzheimer's disease later in life than those who are loners. The brain loves company!

Because stroke is also a leading cause of dementia, it is clear that good cardiovascular health (exercise, low-fat diet, lowering cholesterol) can help prevent this form of dementia. Some research has suggested that the same heart-healthy habits may also help prevent Alzheimer's disease.

Finally, although it will probably not prevent Alzheimer's disease altogether, researchers believe staying intellectually active might delay the onset. Keep doing your crossword puzzles, read books, learn new skills, and expose yourself to new information. It seems to be good for the brain and may prevent or delay the onset of dementia.

How Does a Person with Alzheimer's Disease or Other Dementia Become Part of a Research Study?

Many individuals with dementia and their families maintain an interest in supporting research, either to help the person currently affected or to assist future generations. Most families try to link with one of the national Alzheimer's disease university research centers. There should never be a charge to participate, and an easy-to-understand informed consent form should be made available.

To find a university study, check the websites beginning on page 283 or contact your local Alzheimer's Association or Society. Most of these nonprofit groups maintain ties to area research centers and studies.

Early-Stage and Younger-Onset Alzheimer's Disease

Younger-onset Alzheimer's disease is a term generally applied to individuals diagnosed with the disease before the age of sixty-five. The field previously used the phrase "early onset." We like the new term since it more clearly describes the person and doesn't cause confusion with the term "early stage."

Early-stage Alzheimer's disease describes an individual in any age bracket who has been diagnosed early in the disease process. Stages are fairly arbitrary, but this individual may: have insight about his or her situation; be able to express his or her thoughts; hold down his or her job; verbally express wishes and concerns; live with minimal supervision; and maintain many daily routines. Yet the person may also have noticeable memory lapses and other mishaps.

What Happens at the End?

Alzheimer's disease causes a gradual decline in the body's ability to take care of itself. The disease causes physiological changes to the brain that take a devastating toll on the person, who eventually may be unable to swallow, walk, or manage most or all activities of daily living. Because of this, Alzheimer's disease does eventually take the life of the person. On death certificates, Alzheimer's disease is often listed as a secondary cause of death, with the more immediate cause (typically heart attack, stroke, and pneumonia) listed first. In general, most persons die *with* Alzheimer's disease, not from it.

Discussions around death and dying today involve many ethical issues such as withholding nutrition; use of life-support systems, feeding tubes, or pegs; giving emergency resuscitation; and other issues. Many families also review medications at this time. Does someone need to be on three cardiovascular medications or baby aspirin to prevent heart attack if he or she is in late dementia?

The hospice movement has contributed greatly to the notion that no one should have to experience undue pain or suffering in his or her final days. It is important that you and your family be assertive with the medical community at this difficult time to make your wishes known and to respect the wishes and values of the person with dementia. The next chapter discusses advanced directives, which are documents that allow people to say how they feel about continuing medical treatments should they become gravely ill or incapacitated.

CONCLUSION

The pace of change in dementia research has been rapid. A hopeful time has arrived when more effective treatments and preventive measures are on the horizon. To keep abreast of changes, subscribe to local and national Alzheimer's Association publications and check out reputable websites that have accurate information and are not trying to sell you a product. You may also live close to a university research center that has staff who you can call for information, a newsletter, workshops, or conferences.

We have much to celebrate in terms of progress on research, but one should always be cautious about "breakthrough" news. Science seems often to move "two steps forward, one step back." If you read about something that seems too good to be true, it probably is. If a friend gives you an Internet article or reference about a breakthrough herb, the odds are high that the study being cited was funded by the manufacturer or that the research is not scientifically sound. Yet, breakthroughs do come in unusual ways. All of us should just practice healthy skepticism and be aware that any bona fide breakthrough will quickly be shared with the world.

Best Friends Pointers

- Dementia is an umbrella term for many reversible and irreversible disorders that can cause memory loss and cognitive decline. Alzheimer's is the most common dementia.
- Do your best to stay informed by attending workshops or conferences and by visiting reputable websites.
- Be wary of reported cures and stories that appear too good to be true; they probably are.
- Ask your doctor about current medications that may enhance thinking and memory.

3

WHAT NOW?

Steps to Take After a Diagnosis of Alzheimer's Disease or Other Dementia

In many cases, a diagnosis of Alzheimer's disease or other dementia does not come as a complete surprise. Individuals or families may have suspected or seen problems develop, clipped articles from newspapers and magazines, and read information online. Often, adult children or spouses have pushed the individual to see his or her doctor. Yet when the diagnosis is finally delivered, it still comes as a shock.

What now? This is the time to begin the all-important process of planning ahead, identifying critical services that might help the person, and getting legal and financial matters in order. It is also a time to educate yourself about dementia, to set appropriate expectations for the person, to think about how the disease will change your relationship with the person and your entire family, and to begin to develop a philosophy and plan of care. The Alzheimer's Disease Bill of Rights on page 55 is a starting point for considering the ethical issues surrounding care. This Bill of Rights can also be useful to individuals with Alzheimer's disease as they weigh options and make plans.

The diagnosis can be overwhelming, and you may find yourself wondering how to talk to the person after the diagnosis is made, how to address your own anxieties about dealing with the situation, and how this new awareness affects your finances. Following are some pointers on how to do these things; all of these important steps are within your power to accomplish.

Be Open with the Person About His or Her Situation

Almost all physicians believe that ethically they are required to tell adult patients about their condition or diagnosis, even if it contradicts the wishes of friends and family. Families struggle with this concept, worrying that the diagnosis will be so devastating that the person will be plunged into despair, depression, or even suicide. Thankfully, most of these fears about disclosing the diagnosis are never realized. In fact, the person with dementia may be relieved to know that he or she isn't "crazy" or may simply forget the details of the discussion.

Straight talk and openness offer the opportunity for the person to participate in decision making. Persons in the early stage of Alzheimer's disease or other dementia typically want to maintain independence as much and as long as they can. Examples range from everyday decisions to more profound ones. The person may want to pick out his clothes for the day, order off the menu himself, or decide what time to wake up in the morning. By talking about the diagnosis, the person will also be able to express wishes or make plans for his or her own future. This is a time to encourage life review and reflection and talk about important topics.

An Alzheimer's Disease Bill of Rights

Every person diagnosed with Alzheimer's disease or a related disorder deserves:

To be informed of one's diagnosis.

To have appropriate, ongoing medical care.

To be productive in work and play as long as possible.

To be treated like an adult, not a child.

To have expressed feelings taken seriously.

To be free from psychotropic medications if at all possible.

To live in a safe, structured, and predictable environment.

To enjoy meaningful activities to fill each day.

To be out-of-doors on a regular basis.

To have physical contact, including hugging, caressing, and handholding.

To be with persons who know one's life story, including cultural and religious traditions.

To be cared for by individuals well-trained in dementia care.

From *The Best Friends Approach to Alzheimer's Care*, ©2003, Health Professions Press. Used with permission.

Openness has so much importance. By keeping the diagnosis secret, families profoundly limit their ability to use services and talk to the person, friends, and family about day-to-day care. By talking openly about the disease, you may be surprised to find a silver lining: Your family member may handle the news with more resilience than you might expect.

Deal with Denial

Many times the person or his or her care partners fall into denial immediately after hearing the diagnosis. One husband, for instance, proceeded with naming his wife with Alzheimer's disease as the executor of their will because, as he said, "I didn't want to hurt her feelings!" In the short run, denial is healthy in that it helps the care partner and person cope with the shock of the diagnosis. In the long run, however, denial is harmful. A care partner who holds onto denial too strongly and too long becomes isolated from friends and family and often underutilizes services or fails to use services at all.

When a person or care partner is in denial, the best remedy is often time and patience. Confrontation, arguing, and overexplaining rarely work. It's a good idea to regularly expose this person to information about dementia. Attending a workshop, conference, or support group can be helpful.

Family meetings are another good way to help one another overcome denial, share information, and develop an action plan. Whenever possible, have an outside facilitator—perhaps someone from the local Alzheimer's Association, a trusted religious advisor, a social worker or counselor, an attorney, or staff member from a day center—come to the family meeting. A skilled facilitator will work to get all of the issues on the table and will encourage everyone in the family to speak up. A family meeting can also provide a good forum for crafting a plan for the future and deciding on individual responsibilities to share the caregiving load, which helps preserve family relationships.

Be Open with Others About Your Family Situation

The words of the poet John Donne—"No man is an island"—are important to remember. Care partners who isolate themselves have a more difficult time. Family and friends will eventually recognize that something is wrong. Get ahead of the curve and speak openly about your situation now. It is comforting to know that the stigma surrounding Alzheimer's disease is diminishing rapidly. When families attend support groups for the first time, they are often surprised to find people they know, maybe even neighbors. Being open about a loved one's diagnosis and the family's goals to provide home care can allow friends and neighbors to offer assistance and lead to an expanded support network.

Get Legal and Financial Affairs in Order

The person with Alzheimer's disease will gradually be unable to make important legal and financial decisions (sadly, this may already be the case). Following are four of the most important legal arrangements to make:

1. Wills and trusts should be written or revised and filed in a place where they can be located when needed.
2. A trusted party should be given a durable power of attorney (DPOA) for finances. A durable power of attorney survives a

person's incapacity. It allows care partners to handle financial affairs and make important decisions. The primary care partner should also designate a trusted individual with a DPOA in case the care partner becomes sick or incapacitated while still responsible for the person.

3. A healthcare Power of Attorney allows you to name someone who can get access to your health records, talk to health care providers, or advocate for you if you are not able to. This is an important document for care partners to organize as soon as possible after a diagnosis; not having one can make it hard to talk to doctors and healthcare providers and arrange for other services, such as a placement in assisted-living memory care.
4. Everyone should have a "living will," also known as an advance directive. This document tells friends and family your wishes regarding end-of-life care (for example, if you want to be resuscitated or have a feeding tube under certain circumstances or not at all). Sometimes this document is combined with, or is part of, the power of attorney for health care discussed above.

Consulting a legal advisor about your situation is essential after a diagnosis of Alzheimer's or dementia: Sometimes simple, inexpensive steps taken early can save thousands of dollars later. Consult a reputable elder-law attorney or local social service agency for help. If you cannot afford legal assistance, contact a local senior service agency or your Alzheimer's Association for a referral to a nonprofit legal service program (many of which are free or low cost).

Be very cautious if the person is still handling his or her own money. Judgment is impaired by dementia and even the most financially savvy individual can be taken advantage of by unscrupulous salespeople or even "bad apple" family members. If the person is making bad financial decisions and refuses to give up control or accept help, the family may have to turn to the courts for the appointment of a conservator. This can sometimes be avoided by financial DPOA documents. Be vigilant! Financial abuse of elders is a growing problem.

Make a Financial Plan for Health Care Services

One significant problem facing families is the enormous rise in healthcare and long-term care costs. Many prescriptions can run $150 or more per month. Residential care programs can cost $50,000 a year or more. These costs can threaten a family's financial security, perhaps even wipe out the nest egg parents had hoped to leave for children and grandchildren.

Typical costs include use of adult day center care, in-home care, medications, and residential care (although not everyone with dementia ends up in residential care). Many care partners have to give up work opportunities or retire early in order to take over care tasks. This can ultimately damage their finances and retirement options. A 2012 report from the Alzheimer's Association describes the economic costs of Alzheimer's disease and other dementia on families and on our health care system. Care partners in the U.S. provide billions of dollars of informal care, but direct costs for families over the long haul of dementia can reach tens, if not hundreds, of thousands of dollars (http://www.alz.org/downloads/facts_figures_2012.pdf).

Don't give up hope if you have limited finances. Many adult day centers have sliding fee scales or charge reasonable daily fees. You or your loved one may be eligible for various social programs, including

Medicaid or care from the Veterans' Administration. A local senior service agency or your Alzheimer's Association can help you locate affordable, appropriate care. One good source of help is a National Council on Aging program called Benefits Check Up; the website can help you determine if you or a family member is eligible for various benefit programs (www.benefitscheckup.org).

Long-term care insurance pays for many home services, day care visits, and residential care stays. We highly recommend these policies. Unfortunately, once someone is beginning to exhibit signs of dementia, it is too late to buy such a policy because the person does not pass the required medical examination.

Make a Realistic Assessment of Yourself and Your Community

Before assuming responsibility for caring for someone with dementia, you should first think about your own health, your attitudes about caregiving, your financial resources, and your coping skills. Are you up for the task? There is no shame if your answer is "no." In fact, realizing this can do the person a great service because you will be able to arrange a caregiving situation that will be more optimal.

Next, see whether your community is resource rich or resource poor in elder or dementia services. Are you in a rural setting where transportation is difficult? Is there a day center nearby? Are there nearby support groups? If your community does not have these services, you can consider moving (take your time with this decision, though—conventional wisdom dictates that care partners not make drastic changes to their living situations right after a diagnosis). Better yet, become an advocate for change, raise awareness, and organize services to help yourself, friends, and neighbors who are dealing with Alzheimer's disease.

If your community does have resources, do not wait too long to take advantage of them. Families often wait until the person has deteriorated beyond the family's ability to provide good care. Family members then find themselves stymied by waiting lists and are forced to make important decisions under pressure. Planning ahead, whenever possible, is important.

Make a Realistic Assessment of Your Loved One with Dementia

As a care partner, you need to set expectations of the person that are neither too high nor too low. If you set your expectations too high ("Dad can still pay his bills if he just tries harder; he can finish that chore on his own, don't help him"), you risk failure and frustration on the part of the person with dementia. There are also safety concerns. If a care partner sets expectations too high and leaves the person alone, the result could be a fire if the stove is left on or a flood if the bath overflows.

Look for Remaining Strengths

Is the person:

Friendly, happy being with others?
Kind, considerate, compassionate?
Affectionate, both giving and receiving affection?
Musical?
Humorous, enjoys the humor of others?

Good with children?

Helpful, wanting to do things for others?

Energetic, a hard worker?

Creative?

Religious and/or spiritual?

If you have answered "yes" to any of these questions, if you have found some remaining strengths, try to engage the person in the following activities:

Reminisce about work, early childhood, or other past events.

Spend time outdoors, take walks.

Do yard work, gardening, or household chores.

Ask the person to teach another an old skill.

Spend time with children or enjoy a pet.

Give lots of hugs.

Read a newspaper or thumb through magazines.

Talk about what he or she has valued most.

Linger over breakfast or coffee.

Attend a worship service, sing a familiar hymn or religious song.

If you set expectations too low ("Dad can't do anything; don't even try"), the person becomes bored and disconnected from life and his or her failures are magnified. With coaching and encouragement, people with dementia can often still help with household chores, brushing the dog, sorting a drawer, tasting the soup, completing a drawing, and other life-enhancing activities.

You will also want to ask yourself questions such as: How is this person's overall health—vision, hearing, and mobility? How much has the dementia progressed? How bad is his or her memory? How limited has the person's ability to communicate or to understand directions become? As difficult as it is to see your loved one decline, try to think about the person's remaining strengths and abilities. "Look for Remaining Strengths" on page 61 can help you begin thinking about these preserved abilities.

Work to Preserve, or Even Enhance, Family Relationships

Alzheimer's disease and other dementia rarely leave a family unchanged. They typically either bring family members closer together or push them apart. Family members should discuss their expectations with one another and ask themselves what kind of relationship they want with each other in the future.

Common problems include:

- one family member becoming disproportionately responsible for care responsibilities
- emergence of unresolved family conflicts
- sibling rivalries
- conflicts over money and use of resources
- disagreements about decisions
- disappointments over broken commitments.

Attending support groups, obtaining family counseling or mediation, and making a thoughtful plan for the future are strategies to help prevent or solve family conflicts.

Safe Return Program

The Alzheimer's Association MedicAlert™ Safe Return Program

Almost everyone with dementia is at risk for a wandering incident because it is easy for the person to become confused about time and place. A person may forget common landmarks and get lost during a walk around the neighborhood or decide he or she is late for work and leave the house.

If wandering is a concern, make use of the Alzheimer's Association's MedicAlert™ Safe Return Program (www.alz.org/safereturn), a nationwide program in the United States that provides an engraved identification bracelet or necklace, iron-on clothing labels, and other materials that provide personal identification for the person. For a one-time startup fee and a modest annual charge, the program can be helpful in a medical emergency or wandering incident. The MedicAlert™ Safe Return program maintains a 24-hour telephone line. If a person wanders and is found, at any time of day, the identification materials can be used to return him or her to home. The program registration requires a photograph of the person that can be sent electronically to first responders if the person unexpectedly disappears.

One advantage of the Safe Return program is that it also covers care partners in case of an emergency. If the care partner is registered and becomes sick or disabled, the first responders have a tool to recognize that the individual has important caregiving responsibilities and can take appropriate steps to ensure everyone's safety.

Make the Environment Simple and Safe

Simplifying the household can make the everyday job of caregiving much easier. If the person struggles with decisions about what to wear, he or she should not maintain a closet full of outfits from which to choose. If the person is unsteady on his or her feet, then furniture, area rugs, or objects that clutter pathways should be removed and grab bars should be installed in bathrooms to help prevent falls. Improving lighting in main living areas is important, particularly because many older people have vision problems in addition to dementia.

Also, assess and adjust your home's safety by looking at locks, fencing, access to the stove, water temperature, and the accessibility of toxic products. It is always a good idea to make extra sets of keys in case they are lost. Give an extra set to a trusted neighbor, friend, or family member. Or buy a lock box that stashes a key and attaches to a front porch rail or pipe. (A lock box can also help first responders and save the front door from being broken down!)

Continue to Be Part of the Community

Going out for breakfast, enjoying a concert in the park, taking a drive, attending a worship service, and doing other things outside of the house are all part of life and should be incorporated into your daily routine whenever possible. These activities benefit both the person with Alzheimer's and his or her care partner, particularly when the care partner chooses things he or she enjoys.

Success often requires some creativity on your part. If the regular worship service is too crowded for the person to enjoy, attend a different service. Going out to breakfast at 10 AM instead of the busy hours from 7 AM to 9 AM may be less stressful. You can inform the restaurant staff of the person's diagnosis so they can greet him or her with a warm smile and be more patient with the menu order.

Staying socially engaged is important for all of us. If the person with dementia can still volunteer at an animal shelter, read a book to children, visit a local art museum, or go to a local coffee shop it adds value and meaning to life, raises self-esteem, and fights depression.

CONCLUSION

The most important thing to do after a family member receives a diagnosis of Alzheimer's disease or dementia may be the most difficult for some—acceptance of the situation. Acceptance is fostered by understanding the emotions and feelings of the person with dementia and developing empathy for his or her plight. When a care partner can accept the disease as real, the next steps toward becoming a Best Friend become easier.

Making both a short- and a long-range plan is an important and positive step. A husband will not be able to stop the progress of his wife's dementia, but he can take care of legal and financial planning. A son may not be able to bring back his mother's gift for language, but he can find a day center with a good music program for her. A wife may not be able to alleviate her husband's anxiety, but she can go to a support group to deal with her own worries and concerns so she can more calmly address his.

You are really at a fork in the road. You can choose to go it alone or choose a path that will benefit you, your friends, your family, and the person with dementia.

Best Friends Pointers

- Don't keep the diagnosis a secret. Talk about it with the person and share the news about your situation with friends and family.
- Give a high priority to legal and financial affairs so that you have the tools you need to travel the caregiving journey.
- Take a good look at your ability to be the primary care partner. Who can help you? What services can you use to help your situation?
- Don't get overwhelmed or wait too long to use services.
- Take one day at a time.

II

THE BEST FRIENDS APPROACH

4

A NEW START

The Art of Friendship

Alzheimer's disease and other dementia change us all. Because of the associated memory loss and confusion, your mother, father, sister, brother, husband, wife, or partner may no longer know you or understand his or her relationship to you. Many friends and family members are confused, frustrated, sad, or even angry about these losses. Your mother may have always been your closest confidante and strongest supporter; now, she does not recognize you. A spouse whom you counted on for many years to balance the checkbook, pay bills, file the income taxes, or cook three meals a day is no longer able to do these things. Your longtime neighbor famous for her home baking now forgets your name and burns her cakes in the oven. As a result, your relationship with the person changes whether you like it or not.

Adopting a Best Friends approach can have a powerful impact on the person with dementia. When you rethink, or recast, your relationship to an individual with dementia and become the person's Best Friend, the person feels you are on his or her side. This can reduce behaviors that are challenging and foster cooperation. In addition, friendship helps evoke some of the social graces or learned manners of the person with dementia. It helps the person with dementia operate at his or her best.

Adopting a Best Friends approach can help diminish the pain and loss you feel about your situation. It can restore a sense of fun, support good conversation, help you overcome the bad days, and teach you ways to encourage activity. Dementia has changed the relationship you have always had with your family member or friend; memories are lost and routines disrupted—but a Best Friends approach helps to build a new kind of relationship that can also be healing. "Mom is now my friend," one care partner told us. "She doesn't exactly remember who I am, but we are having more fun than ever as best girlfriends."

Because of its pioneering use of the Best Friends approach, the Best Friends Day Center in Lexington, Kentucky (formerly named "Helping Hand"), has become one of the most admired adult day programs in the United States. Many individuals who attend this dementia-specific center have been considered difficult and challenging by their own family care partners. Yet at this day program, because the staff and volunteers are acting as friends, all persons thrive. Families can have similar success using the Best Friends approach at home.

Rather than staying in a state of despair, care partners can learn to work through the pain and focus on gaining maximum value from the present; caregiving is transformed from a terrible burden to a job that becomes meaningful and satisfying. The process changes from a series of failures to a series of successes, turning a "no" into a "yes." Recasting this relationship to become a Best Friend does not mean taking away love or loving the person with dementia any less. It simply means approaching the relationship differently.

One son attending an Alzheimer's conference told us that he had always had a troublesome relationship with his father—so bad, in fact, that he ran away from home at age sixteen. He now cares for his father full time and says they have never been closer. They take a daily walk together, have an evening scotch and soda, and watch the grandchildren play soccer. They have found that they now enjoy each other's company. Because the father has forgotten much of the past and is often unsure of his relationship with his son, the son has realized that he, too, must let go of past slights and injustices. "What's the point of me dwelling on it?" the son asks. "What's past is past."

Like many care partners, the son never dreamed he would be in the position of taking care of his father, a father whom he admits disliking for much of his life. However, this family's approach to Alzheimer's care has helped heal not only the son's relationship with his father, but also wounds he has carried inside himself.

Being a Best Friend is not just about altruism. Care partners who recast their relationships take advantage of the principles of friendship to gain new ideas for handling day-to-day care in a more natural, positive way; prevent problems before they happen; form a new relationship with a loved one based on getting the most out of every day; and replace the stress and strain of caregiving with satisfaction. The following are the key ingredients for success:

What Is a Best Friend?

FRIENDS KNOW EACH OTHER'S PERSONALITY AND HISTORY

A Best Friend becomes the person's memory.

A Best Friend is sensitive to the person's traditions.

A Best Friend respects the person's personality, moods, and problem-solving style.

FRIENDS DO THINGS TOGETHER

A Best Friend initiates activities.

A Best Friend encourages the person to enjoy the simple things in life.

A Best Friend enjoys activities with the person with dementia.

A Best Friend involves the person in chores.

A Best Friend ties activities into the person's past skills and interests.

A Best Friend remembers to celebrate special occasions.

FRIENDS COMMUNICATE

A Best Friend listens.

A Best Friend fills in the blanks.

A Best Friend asks questions that are easily answered.

A Best Friend recognizes the importance of nonverbal communication.

A Best Friend gently encourages participation in conversations.

FRIENDS BUILD SELF-ESTEEM

A Best Friend gives compliments often.

A Best Friend carefully asks for advice or opinions.

A Best Friend always offers encouragement.

A Best Friend offers congratulations.

FRIENDS LAUGH TOGETHER OFTEN

A Best Friend tells jokes and funny stories.

A Best Friend takes advantage of spontaneous fun.

A Best Friend uses self-deprecating humor often.

FRIENDS ARE EQUALS

A Best Friend does not talk down to the person.

A Best Friend works to help the person "save face."

A Best Friend does not assume a supervisor role.

A Best Friend recognizes that learning is a two-way street.

FRIENDS WORK AT THE RELATIONSHIP

A Best Friend is not overly sensitive.

A Best Friend does more than half the work.

A Best Friend builds a trusting relationship.

A Best Friend shows affection often.

FRIENDS KNOW EACH OTHER'S PERSONALITY AND HISTORY

Typically, people become friends because they have something in common; perhaps they graduated from the same high school or college or both enjoy Monday night football. As the friendship grows, they learn more about each other—how many brothers and sisters each has, their birthdays and birthplaces, cultural and religious traditions, hobbies, and special achievements. As much as we think we know our friends, there are often surprises. Perhaps it turns out a friend once thought to be strictly a country music fan has a passion for opera.

Friends also become good judges of each other's moods and personalities. A friend develops a sense of timing, such as where and when not to tease someone. Friends even begin to understand each other's problem-solving style, knowing when a word of advice is welcome and when it may be resented.

A Best Friend Becomes the Person's Memory

A Best Friend should bring up as much as possible about the person in order to offer cues and reminders of his or her previous achievements. If the person has early-stage Alzheimer's, work with him or her to develop a Life Story (see page 101). Even if you think you know all about a parent or sibling, you will be surprised to see from his or her perspective which experiences stand out.

When friends or family members spend time with Mary Edith Engle, they know that they can always bring a smile to her face when they remind her of her extraordinary life and accomplishments, notably as one of the elite female pilots during World War II, when she was a member of the Women's Air Force Service Pilots (WASP). "You're very petite to have flown those big B-29 bombers. Are you just kidding us? Did you really fly those planes?" a friend may ask. "Sure did," Mary Edith replies.

Mary Edith has been inducted into the Kentucky Aviation Hall of Fame. When young women volunteers talk with her at the day center, they often gain new respect for her as a trailblazing woman for her times.

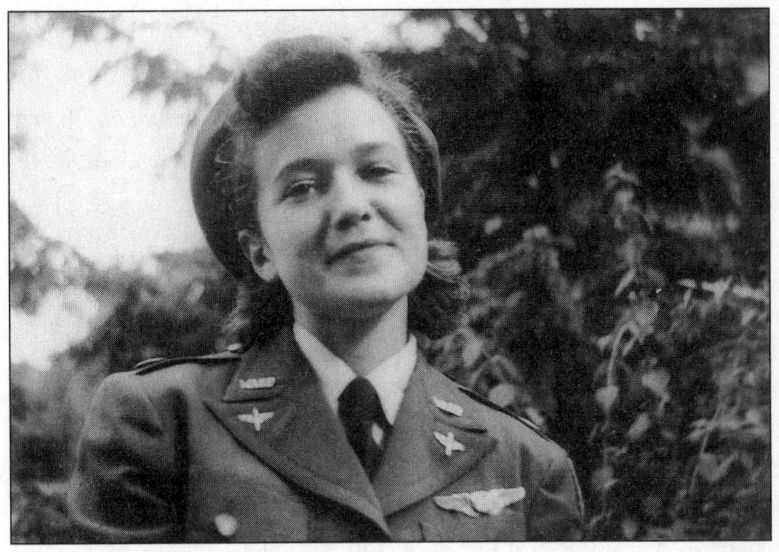

Mary Edith Engle in her WASP uniform, 1944.

A Best Friend Is Sensitive to the Person's Traditions

Even late in the illness, the person often retains his or her values and traditions. Religious traditions and faith, for example, are deep-seated, and knowing a person's beliefs can be important in providing quality care. Knowing this also helps a Best Friend understand why individuals sometimes do the things they do.

Leota Kilkenny always had a good appetite and enjoyed lunch at the day center she attended at a local church. One day, she refused to eat her lunch, saying, "I cannot. I must not now." She became agitated after several attempts had been made to encourage her to eat, so the staff let her skip the meal. When her daughter, Ann, picked her up that day she solved the mystery by saying that while they were driving to the day center she had told her mother they were going to the program "at the Church." Ann told the staff, "Mother is Catholic and must have thought she was going to her church and would be taking communion. In her tradition, you do not eat within an hour before receiving communion."

This is an example of one way that a deeply felt tradition, even one that cannot be expressed in words, can affect daily care.

A Best Friend Respects the Person's Personality, Moods, and Problem-Solving Style

Personalities and problem-solving styles do sometimes change with the onset of dementia, but the underlying attitudes and styles usually remain. For example, a person who always coped well with adversity may bring some of this resiliency to living with dementia. A person who has always been a "take-charge" individual or in a position of authority generally does not like being told what to do.

Marydean Evans always told her friends and family that she was not a morning person and could be in a bad mood until midmorning. When she attended a day center, the sensitive staff and volunteers empathized and greeted her each morning with a remark such as, "Marydean, I know you're not a morning person. Would some coffee help? How about five cups?"

Knowing Marydean's quirks, a Best Friend would never press her to be involved in day center activities too early in the morning, respecting her desire to wake up slowly over some hot coffee. The teasing remark about "five cups" tickled Marydean's sense of humor.

FRIENDS DO THINGS TOGETHER

Friendships often form based upon mutual activities; you may meet someone on a hike or at a coffee shop, hit it off, and become great friends. Friendships are sustained when you continue to "do things together." When you stop doing things together, friendships flounder and relationships suffer.

A Best Friend Initiates Activities

Because the person often loses the ability to initiate activities or to fully understand a request, it generally is a mistake to ask the person if he or she wants to do something. The answer will often be "no." Instead, a Best Friend could say, for example, "I would like to take a walk. Come on, join me! It's great to exercise with you."

"Come on, Pops! Let's go for a drive," said Riki, the son of Mas Matsumura, who sensed just the right time to initiate one of his father's favorite activities. "Pops loved riding shotgun in the car. He keeps time to '50s music from a CD and enjoys seeing and commenting on cars and people along the way."

Riki spent many hours with his father every day. He knew that when he initiated activities that his dad enjoyed, such as taking a walk, being with children, watching old movies, or going for a drive, the day went better for both of them.

A Best Friend Encourages the Person to Enjoy the Simple Things in Life

Simple things are often the best things in Alzheimer's care. For example, it can be pleasurable for both of you to browse in a bookstore. Perhaps you'll discuss seeing a teenager with green hair, have fun looking through art books, or find a cozy corner with two comfortable chairs. This activity might not work for every situation; a person might become agitated by a large crowd. If you are unsure, take a trial run—keep the visit short, and go when the store is less crowded. You know your loved one best. If he or she is getting restless, it is time to go home.

Serge Gajardo and his wife found pleasure in a simple activity: they often stopped by garage sales. Serge had collected wood carvings and art from all over the world, and he still enjoyed browsing for treasures and irresistible bargains.

Silence is also part of any friendship. Sometimes it is nice simply to sit in a comfortable chair and watch the world go by together or to watch friends or family play a game or watch television. The person can still feel a sense of involvement and security by being in the presence of others.

A Best Friend Enjoys Activities with the Person with Dementia

It is difficult to imagine life without things to do. Most of us like to stay engaged with family and friends in a great variety of ways. Persons with dementia are no different. They long to be in the flow of life and continue the things that have given them meaning.

Tom Meyers is a volunteer at the Best Friends Day Center and Bob Steele is a program participant. They are always very engaged. They both served in the military, one in the Navy and the other in the Army. They banter back and forth about which branch of service is most important. They both have traveled extensively because of their service experience as well as for pleasure. They enjoy looking at maps to locate their favorite spots and to dream of their next trip. Tom and Bob are both members of the Civil War Roundtable, a study group in the community. They enjoy poring over the notes from the Roundtable meetings and discussing them afterward.

Tom enjoys being with Bob as much as Bob enjoys being with Tom. Activities build better relationships and add fun and variety to our daily lives.

A Best Friend Involves the Person in Chores

Even with limited skills, the person can often help with daily chores, such as drying the dishes or stacking the newspapers to recycle. The key to all of these activities is to get the person involved, to encourage him or her to be a part of life. This also connects the person with his or her care partner—it is satisfying to do a project together.

The Gajardos were together at home for ten years after Sergio ("Serge"), an executive for a large company, was diagnosed with Alzheimer's disease. Little by little many things they once enjoyed were no longer possible. Yet his wife, Gertrude, found that Serge could still enjoy many daily chores, such as chopping up vegetables for a stir-fry dinner they could then enjoy.

Serge felt competent and successful when he helped to prepare the evening meal. One reason why this activity was successful is that it had a clear purpose and outcome (preparing dinner and enjoying it). As a Best Friend, Gertrude could praise Serge for the delicious dinner and thank him for his hard work.

A Best Friend Ties Activities into the Person's Past Skills and Interests

Past skills and special interests often remain intact well into the advent of Alzheimer's disease. This is why it's important to know a person's special interests; perhaps he or she can still pursue these interests, particularly with some help and assistance.

Tap Steven has always loved writing and poetry. Despite the onset of Alzheimer's disease, Tap still writes, attends classes, and occasionally teaches. He and his wife, Frankie, are proud that a number of his poems have been published in Alzheimer's newsletters and journals.

Because people like Tap have led such full, rich lives, the possibilities for activities linked to past skills are unlimited.

A Best Friend Remembers to Celebrate Special Occasions

The ritual of a birthday party, anniversary celebration, Veterans' Day parade, or other long-held traditions can bring back many positive memories for the person. Special occasions can be celebrated throughout the year, making a big day out of a birthday or other family event.

Phil and Karen Zwicke renewed their marriage vows after many years of marriage. Surrounded by friends and family, the couple enjoyed the afternoon, including champagne and wedding cake. Phil, then fifty-two, had been open with others about his diagnosis of Alzheimer's disease; both of them were determined to keep him active and enjoying life as long as possible.

Phil enjoyed these simple life celebrations, just as he enjoyed being at one with nature in his beautiful home of Santa Barbara.

FRIENDS COMMUNICATE

The best friendships often involve a lot of talking. Whether it is on the telephone or over the office water cooler, friends generally love to swap stories, gossip, share ideas, send e-mails and instant messages to each other, and confide in one another. Friends are also there to listen to each other, in good and bad times.

A Best Friend Listens

In dementia care, it is important to try to be there for the person when he or she wants to talk about important feelings. Individuals with Alzheimer's disease should be given time to offer their feelings or ideas. Sometimes patience is rewarded with an insight.

Maria Scorsone has spoken three languages in her lifetime: Italian as a child, Spanish when she lived in Argentina, and English after she moved to the United States. She now often mixes the three languages. Her in-home aides became her Best Friends by listening to Maria's words very carefully. When the aides cannot follow the exact words, they can usually still understand her by listening to the tone of her voice and watching her facial expression and other body language.

Maria's gift with languages allowed her to be a teacher to the staff who enjoyed learning words and phrases from languages they didn't speak.

A Best Friend Fills in the Blanks

People with dementia begin to lose the structure of their sentences and language. When you can provide clues and cues, communication can vastly improve. Sometimes even filling in the blanks by supplying one or two words keeps the dialogue going.

Edna Edwards loves to converse but has major difficulty finding the right words. When Edna says "Those little ones, I miss them . . . at the school . . ." her Best Friend says "Picadome School?" Edna can continue, "Picadome, that's my school!"

Conversation can continue about early childhood days, her teaching, and her schoolchildren, all because her Best Friend brought up some familiar names of people, places, and things in Edna's life.

A Best Friend Asks Questions That Are Easily Answered

The person may become easily frustrated if asked questions to which he or she does not know the answer.

When Evelyn Talbott, a retired librarian, returned from a vacation, she would have been frustrated if someone had asked her to recall, "Where did you go on vacation?" or "What was the name of the beach?" Instead, a friend asked skillfully, "Did you and your husband, Bob, have a good time watching those big waves on the ocean?"

When her Best Friend provided some details within the question, it triggered memories and allowed Evelyn to share her joy from her vacation and participate in the conversation.

A Best Friend Recognizes the Importance of Nonverbal Communication

Because verbal skills are diminished, body language becomes very important in dementia care. A Best Friend should greet the person warmly, smile broadly, and hold out a hand. The handshake still holds special meaning with older people who remember a time when everyone in polite company would shake hands. Almost always, the person will respond with a handshake. A mutual handshake is the beginning of a bond, a deep-rooted symbol that one is a friend, not a foe. Talking with your hands can also be effective. Gestures such as tapping the seat on a chair can help the person get the message to sit down.

Because of Mary Burmaster's hearing loss, body language was especially effective for a day center volunteer relating to her. After making eye contact, the volunteer would smile and say, "Mary, lunch is ready." The volunteer would then touch her gently on the shoulder, pat her hand, and guide her to the table.

A Best Friend's gentle touch spoke volumes.

A Best Friend Gently Encourages Participation in Conversations

It is important to include the person in conversations as much as possible. Broad, open-ended questions ("Tell me about . . ."; "What do you think about . . .") that touch on the person's life experience can be particularly effective.

There is so much in Jim Holloway's life to talk about: fishing with his uncle, raising German shepherd dogs, collecting yo-yos, studying great artists and their works, enjoying classical music, teaching theology, visiting Pompeii, attending Yale University, working on old cars, being a medic on a troop ship during WWII, and much more.

All of this stays tucked away until a Best Friend gently encourages conversation by saying, "Tell me about . . ."

The Art of Friendship Comes Naturally

At a skilled nursing home we spoke to a diverse group of staff—many of whom spoke English as a second language—about the Best Friends approach. Instead of giving the staff lists of things to do (and not do), we talked about friendship and Alzheimer's care and did an exercise that can be very helpful to you as you support the person in your life with dementia. We first asked participants to name a close friend and say why they are friends. Here are some of the answers:

Maria: She is a good listener
My mother: She's always there for me
Mike: Laughter
Tony: Nonjudgmental
My sister: She knows me so well; we know what each other is thinking
Jackson: Loving
Mia: Honest feedback
Joe: Supportive

We then asked the staff to think about the residents with dementia and whether they thought those persons would respond to some of these characteristics embodied by good friendship. "Yes," the staff answered.

We then asked the staff how a friend could help a resident with dementia in the following scenarios. Here are some of their answers:

The resident seems upset, agitated:	Give her a hug. Ask her what's wrong. Spend some time with her. Check to see if she is physically okay. Sing a song together. Offer a compliment about her pretty pink sweater.
The person is pacing:	Walk with her. Ask her if she needs some help. Tell a funny joke.
The person won't come to an activity he or she usually enjoys:	Tell her we need her. Remind her about it, but gently. Don't bug her and let her decide.
The person is angry:	Tell her you'll look into the problem. Back off for a while. No big deal; I get angry now and then too.

By understanding these concepts—that persons with dementia are just like our own friends with similar needs and feelings—the staff could now stop, look, and listen when problems were brewing and ask themselves, "What would a friend do?" or "How can I be a Best Friend?" This helped them be more successful at work. Being a friend comes naturally, and the elements are simple to put into practice.

Try the above exercise at home. Ask yourself how you can be a Best Friend to Mom if she is upset or angry, frustrated, or not wanting to go out. The Best Friends approach can lead you to new ideas for success.

FRIENDS BUILD SELF-ESTEEM

A good friendship brings out the best in each person. It involves a mutual support system, with each giving the other constructive criticism and feedback as well as unconditional support. Friends also look at strengths more than weaknesses. Self-esteem is built when friends give a compliment, remain loyal, stay in touch, and tell us how important we are to them.

A Best Friend Gives Compliments Often

Telling a person "You look nice today" or "You really did a good job gardening" builds self-esteem. A compliment also can "disarm" the person who is having a bad day or bad moment. The compliment distracts the person, moving him or her away from the problem or concern.

Ruby Mae Morris loved pretty clothes. Compliments for Ruby Mae such as "You are pretty as a picture," "You are all dolled up today, ready for a party," or "That pretty blue dress matches your pretty blue eyes" made her beam. The good feeling she got from the compliments seemed to linger throughout her day.

Recognition in the form of a compliment can be so easy with such big returns. The emotion provided by compliments lasts long after the words are forgotten.

A Best Friend Carefully Asks for Advice or Opinions

Another way to show a person that he or she is valued is by asking for an opinion. The question should not be about the national debt or foreign trade. Instead, you could ask, "I didn't have a chance to look in the mirror today. Do you think my tie matches my shirt?" This could lead to a lengthy discussion about fabrics, textures, colors, changing widths of ties, and perhaps even the need for a new wardrobe.

"What do you think about Mexico, Mother? Do you think it would be a fun place to visit?" Emma Simpson likes it when her daughter Patricia asks her opinion about a future trip.

Even though Emma can no longer travel, she enjoys the fact that Patricia values her opinion. A question like this allows mother and daughter to look at travel brochures together, discuss clothing and the weather, and even talk about what kind of food tourists might eat in Mexico. Like most mothers, Emma is thrilled when her daughter comes to her for advice.

A Best Friend Offers Encouragement

People with Alzheimer's disease need as much encouragement as possible, in many forms. Sometimes it is to encourage individuals by reminding them of their value as friends: "You add so much to my life" or "We're just like sisters." The person can also be encouraged to attempt a particular task, especially a task that seems possible to accomplish. A Best Friend might say, "I could use your help in putting this puzzle together. Would you sit by me and help out?"

A beautiful scarf, creatively displayed to complement her outfit, was Edna Carroll Greenwade's hallmark. One day the director of the day center brought a collection of scarves and encouraged Edna Carroll to show everyone how to wear them. Edna beamed as she helped each participant tie her scarf and, as the fashion show of scarves passed by her for inspection, she exclaimed, "I'm so glad to be of help!"

Often, gentle encouragement is all that is needed to practice an old skill.

A Best Friend Offers Congratulations

In dementia care, the person should be congratulated often for small and big successes.

When Edna Edwards's granddaughter was a finalist in the Miss Kentucky beauty pageant, the day center volunteers said with excitement, "Edna, congratulations on your granddaughter's winning the Miss Kentucky beauty pageant; Mary Dudley must have gotten her good looks from you!" Edna would often respond, "You know it!"

A person can also be congratulated for a current personal or family achievement or for something in the past. Perhaps someone like Edna has been a beauty queen in her own right!

FRIENDS LAUGH TOGETHER

Humor is a powerful element in all relationships. Humor helps people enjoy shared experiences, relieves tension, and brings people together. Many researchers have also confirmed that laughter has positive physiological effects, boosting the immune system and lowering blood pressure.

A Best Friend Tells Jokes and Funny Stories

Even the corniest joke can evoke big laughs from someone with dementia. Funny stories are also popular, particularly ones involving either the care partner or the person. For example, a Best Friend might say, "I still haven't forgiven you for eating the last piece of grandmother's pumpkin pie that Thanksgiving." Don't forget that the person can sometimes remember or tell a great story or joke.

In spite of the fact that he had had a series of strokes, Jerry Ruttenberg retained his great sense of humor. When a volunteer in the day center handed him corn on the cob, he said loudly, "Oh, shucks." Another time, in answer to the serious question, "How do sand dollars reproduce?" he quipped, "They give birth to baby dimes."

It is a running joke in some friendships: "Not that story again, I've heard it before!" Yet in dementia care, a story that is repeated often can be a favorite with the person. It may be that they are simply not remembering hearing it before. More likely, they connect with the smiles, laughter, and joy associated with the story.

A Best Friend Takes Advantage of Spontaneous Fun

Things happen spontaneously that are often humorous for the person and the people around him or her. Laughter can come from watching staff at a nursing home chase a pet rabbit that has gotten free from its cage. Fun can come in many ways:

Riki took advantage of spontaneous moments while caring for his dad, Mas. "Pops loved to laugh at pratfalls and physical humor. Every chance I got I faked bumping my head against a wall or tripping over my feet. At times he caught me faking it, but other times he laughed hysterically. Pops also loved to rhyme and laugh at language used awkwardly or uniquely. He continued to be witty and clever and loved spontaneous humor in people and situations.

There is spontaneous fun all around us free for the taking to help lighten the losses of dementia.

A Best Friend Uses Self-Deprecating Humor Often

Friends are not afraid to be the butt of their own jokes. Embarrassing moments happen to all of us, but are a particular concern of people with dementia. When a person can't find his glasses, a helpful response from a Best Friend might be, "I looked all over for my glasses last week and then found them—right on my nose."

The spotlight at the day center was on Marydean Evans as she demonstrated the steps to the waltz. The group was enjoying the occasion when suddenly Marydean began looking for something to show the group. She was sure that she had it when she came to the program that morning: "I'm always losing my things, and I wanted to show it to everyone." In keeping with the celebratory mood, her Best Friend quipped, "I have the same problem sometimes. Good thing my head is securely fastened. I'd lose it too!"

Self-deprecating humor reassures the person that he or she is not the only one in the world who is forgetful. It also diffuses negative situations and helps the person stay in a positive mood. A good self-deprecating remark also allows for laughter to break the tension, for a frown to turn into a smile.

FRIENDS ARE EQUALS

No friendship will survive condescending behavior. Everyone has different strengths and weaknesses, but differences should be celebrated rather than dwelled on.

A Best Friend Does Not Talk Down to the Person

Condescending language is never appropriate in dementia care. Examples of inappropriate language include speaking in an exaggerated, slow, and measured voice; being insensitive; using childish language; being flippant; not giving the person time to respond to a question; asking inappropriate and embarrassing questions; or talking about a person as though he or she were not present.

Rubena Dean enjoyed looking at cards that contained brief biographies of famous women. One day she was trying to recall facts about Helen Keller when she lost her train of thought. A Best Friend felt her pain at not being able to finish and simply said, "I'm sorry."

Rubena's Best Friend did not condescend by trying to negate or dismiss her feelings. Rubena needed her friend to empathize and be supportive.

A Best Friend Works to Help the Person "Save Face"

Many people with dementia remain fiercely independent. The person may still have a lot of pride and be reluctant to accept help or "charity."

When Margaret Brubaker's friends or family visited, they were often concerned that she was not eating well. She was very proud and refused gifts of food, saying that she was not hungry or had "just eaten an enormous meal!" A volunteer took a different approach. During one visit he said, "Margaret, you could do me such a favor. Bananas were on sale this week, and I bought 3 pounds. My wife went to the store separately and bought 3 pounds. We just don't know what to do with all these bananas. It would help us so much if you'd take some off our hands."

Margaret took the bananas with delight because she was doing her friend a favor and her friend was respecting Margaret's dignity.

A Best Friend Does Not Assume a Supervisory Role

Friends generally have a sense of equality between them. The person wants to feel independent. He or she almost always responds negatively to being bossed around.

Edith Hayes was a devoted mother to her daughter Dona and provided loving care during her childhood. When Edith moved in to her daughter's home, Dona had to tread lightly. "Mother could smell being managed a mile away. Being Best Friends worked well for both of us. I liked to provide opportunities for meaningful things for Mother to do on her own or with family and friends. We as a family are still very active in our church, and we often have gatherings of our four generations, and Mother could still function very well in those family settings. We gave each other space by taking advantage of the local adult day center. Mother always liked being in the helping role; she liked helping others in the center."

Dona knew her mother well and let her mother have her say as much as possible.

A Best Friend Recognizes That Learning Is a Two-Way Street

Equality means learning things from each other. Many people with dementia can still share stories from their personal histories, express compassion and concern, or demonstrate old skills and hobbies.

Dicy Jenkins was a walking encyclopedia of information about plants and herbs used for health and healing. She knew how to use juniper berries, ginseng, feverfew, bee pollen, and burdock root for medicinal purposes.

Many of these old remedies now are actually back in style. Her family and friends remained endlessly fascinated by her wealth of knowledge.

FRIENDS WORK AT THE RELATIONSHIP

Every friendship has its difficult moments. Something said is misconstrued, or a friend disappoints us in some fashion. Clearly no friendship will survive a continuing series of disappointments, but Best Friends discuss disagreements and work them out. Good friendships can handle some rough-and-tumble moments, constructive teasing, and high spirits. Good friendships also require work and commitment. Friends need to stay in touch by phone or letter and initiate activities with each other.

A Best Friend Is Not Overly Sensitive

Friends must recognize that problems, when they occur, are normally part of the disease process, not part of the person. Sometimes, inhibitions are reduced by dementia. The person may say some surprising things.

Geri Greenway valued great art, music, stylish clothes, and beautiful jewelry. When a volunteer in the day center program asked Geri what she thought of some new costume jewelry she had brought to the day program to display, Geri replied, "Well, it looks like a bunch of junk to me."

The experience of the volunteer showed. She replied to the group humorously, "Ask a question, and get an answer."

A Best Friend Does More Than Half of the Work

In dementia care, clearly most of the work is done by the friend without dementia. Just as you would give a friend having tough times some latitude, you should do the same or more with the person with dementia.

"Frances kept us all together—me and our four children. She looked after our every need." Her husband, Bill Tatman, praises her for always being there with clean clothes, good food, appointments made, and picnics planned. Now that she can no longer care for herself, he feels that it is their gift to her to be able to care for her every need.

In this case, Bill and the children may be closer to doing 100 percent of the work, but they recognize that it's now their turn to provide loving support and care.

A Best Friend Builds a Trusting Relationship

Building a trusting relationship takes work, but it can be gained when care partners demonstrate confident, consistent, loving care.

Obviously problems do occur, and some individuals with dementia are distrustful of the world. Piece by piece, however, a trusting relationship can be built and maintained (find out more about this in Chapter 7).

Hobert Elam's wife took time each day to do something that he especially enjoyed. One of his pleasures was to walk hand-in-hand on the farm they owned, look at the Angus cattle, or take a drive to explore the familiar countryside where he grew up.

Just being with his wife, exploring familiar territory, and feeling comforted by the familiar helped Hobert feel more safe and secure. It also reinforced a bond of trust between Hobert and his wife. Walking together, they were husband and wife, but also Best Friends.

A Best Friend Shows Affection Often

We know of some long-term care communities and adult day centers that have a "three hugs a day" rule. Best Friends show the person with dementia affection as often as possible in various ways, including giving compliments, holding hands, giving a pat on the back, hugging, and smiling.

Frances Tatman always loved children and couldn't wait to be a grandmother. Hugs and kisses were one thing that she could still give, and she had lots of those for her seven grandchildren. They returned her affection in double doses.

Affection can take many forms. Most people respond to hugs and touch, but not all. Sometimes affection can come from words or just spending time with the person.

CONCLUSION

Friendship is a powerful part of all our lives. You don't need a college degree to understand it. It is multicultural. Some people have dozens of friends; others just have a few. Even a loner is capable of friendship.

Being a Best Friend restores many of the old social graces of the person with dementia. It provides support and reassurance. It gives us tools to handle everyday concerns and problems. It can reduce many challenging behaviors that people with dementia can have. It can help maintain dignity.

There are still plenty of moments of stress and tension in caring for a person with dementia, but a Best Friends approach can also create moments of contentment and joy—in you and in the person. When you rethink or recast your relationship to the person with dementia, when you become a Best Friend, you can become better prepared to cope with the challenges that arise each day or that lie ahead.

Best Friends Pointers

- The person with dementia mixes up relationships. Wife becomes "mother" or "sister." Recasting relationships to be a Best Friend is a life-affirming, positive response and helps care partners overcome their sense of loss.
- Use the elements of good friendship, such as giving compliments and offering encouragement and support, to develop creative responses to challenges and turn a "no" into a "yes."
- Facing so many losses and isolation, what a person with dementia needs is a good friend—a Best Friend.

5

MEMORY MAKING

Honoring a Person's Life Story

Medical science has developed prostheses for people who have lost limbs, techniques to bring back eyesight for people with cataracts, and devices to improve hearing. Although there is no cure yet for people with Alzheimer's disease or other dementia, we do have a method of bringing back memories—a "human" prosthesis—a Best Friend. Best Friends are the memory, the biographers for people with dementia.

This is why it is so important to know and use the Life Story in all aspects of caring for the person with dementia. The person with dementia is forgetting much of his or her past; when we know and use the Life Story it allows us to navigate conversations, recall happy memories, understand triggers for behavior, provide smart distractions or redirections, and create more meaningful activities.

Dorothy Troxel lived with Alzheimer's disease for ten years and maintained her cheerful disposition throughout much of her journey. When she was having a bad day, her husband Fred or son David would offer her a cup of Earl Grey tea with milk, her favorite. This almost always worked its magic, particularly when it led to a discussion about her Canadian and British heritage.

Sometimes knowing just a simple thing like a person's favorite beverage allows you to create a good moment.

The Life Story is also a way of recording one's life achievements. When families come together to create the document, the Life Story can be a healing tool, a life-affirming project that can increase acceptance and bring family members closer together. It's a celebration of someone's life and can be a memento for generations to come.

The idea of writing down this story might seem overwhelming, but it's not. This chapter will provide you with an outline of what to include, and you probably already know much of the specific information you need to create an effective Life Story. This chapter also shows you how to create a practical "bullet card," a simple Life Story card to use in everyday care (see page 115).

Think of yourself as a detective. Collecting and recording information to write a good Life Story can involve solving family mysteries, interviewing distant relatives and friends, reviewing old photographs and clippings, and asking the person for information, if possible.

It is important to begin documenting the Life Story early. This way, the person with dementia can still contribute many of his or her own stories. If too much time has already passed, much information can still be collected from friends and other family members. A good starting point is to think about generational memories or historic or significant cultural events your family member experienced (e.g., World War II, Frank Sinatra, *The Ed Sullivan Show*, the Beatles, the moon landing, the Vietnam War, Watergate). Do your best. With some attention to this project, you will be amazed at how personal history comes to life.

The Life Story can be woven into all aspects of Alzheimer's care. For a template of how this can be done, see the Life Story of Rebecca Matheny Riley (page 123). Within it, we've included notations on the ways it can be used to provide outstanding care and meaningful activities for a person with dementia.

INGREDIENTS OF THE LIFE STORY

If you are creating a comprehensive Life Story for your mother, you need to remember that the audience for the Life Story is larger than just family members. If your mother ever needs in-home help or day center care, or has to move to a residential care community, this story must paint a picture for staff members who will initially not know your mother well. Be sure to include the ingredients that follow.

Childhood

In Alzheimer's care, understanding the person's earliest years is sometimes more important than familiarity with the later years. Many people with dementia recall their childhoods for far longer than their more recent lives, so we want to know as much as possible about this influential time.

- Record the date and place of birth, but do more than simply write down the basics. Get a feel for the atmosphere in which your mother was raised. Was her birthplace rural or urban? Was she raised in a coal camp in Appalachia or in a Park Avenue penthouse? What were the main industries of the town in which she was raised? Did her hometown have any special claim to fame? She might remember her birthplace as the place where the best apples in the United States are grown, where Corningware was invented, or where everyone admired the Eiffel Tower.
- Try to piece together even a simple family tree of your mother's childhood. Include the names of her grandparents, parents, and siblings. Ask whether there were any particularly influential relatives, such as an adored older sister or a grandmother who baked prize-winning apple pies.
- Talk about school. Does your mother remember her first day of school? This is usually a milestone. Was school enjoyable? Was she a good student? Was there a favorite subject or favorite teacher? We remember one woman who took pride in remembering that she was "Miss Seventh-Grade Square Root!"
- Make note of any interesting or unusual occupations. Was she a pastry chef, master gardener, or art curator? Many older people today emigrated or were children of immigrants, and if you don't already know it, it is often meaningful to find out more about a family's early journeys. Sometimes these stories involve high drama—life-threatening escapes from an oppressive country or a difficult voyage on an unsafe boat.
- Ask about happy and sad events. In finding out about any life-defining childhood events, it is important to find happy

childhood experiences, but it's also essential to understand any traumas in order to avoid triggering unhappy memories. Perhaps a defining moment was winning a student-of-the year award or a statewide fishing contest. It can be valuable to know whether your mother had a troubled childhood (e.g., being orphaned at an early age or surviving a wartime childhood or natural disaster such as a flood or fire).

- Get a feel for major geographical moves undertaken in childhood. If your mother was a "military brat," for example, and lived in many towns and cities, this can spark interest.
- Record family names. These often offer opportunities for your mother to comment.

  "I loved my father. His name was Tobe. I named our daughter Toby for him," Willa McCabe explained proudly.

  Henrietta Frazier enjoys sharing the story about her name: "My father died before I was born, so my mother named me Henrietta, for my father. His name was Henry."

You can also comment on interesting names from the past: "Your mother's name was America; isn't that interesting!" Although they are sometimes dreaded and disdained, nicknames are important to record. Many family members, in fact, express surprise and pleasure to discover a secret nickname their mom or dad once had. Also of note are affectionate names your mother may have called her parents—Mama, Mother, Ma, Pa, Daddy, or Father.

- Learn your mother's favorite childhood activities, hobbies, and games. Sports certainly played a big role for many people; playground games can be recalled and even reenacted. More serious recreational activities, such as playing a musical instrument or collecting stamps and coins, can also be part of a comprehensive Life Story.

- Have her recall pets. Memories of pets are often vivid and pleasurable. Was there a special cat or dog in Mother's childhood, perhaps a black cat named Midnight or a collie just like Lassie? A person may even have had a pet deer on an Idaho ranch. People who grew up in rural areas might recall memories of winning a ribbon for a prize animal at a state fair or of a pig that the family loved too much to eat.

Adolescence

Adolescence is considered one of the most influential life stages. Key life events during this time can include graduating from junior and senior high, dating, buying a first car, and getting a first job. Adolescence is also a time when children gain greater independence from parents—the first steps to adulthood.

Recipe for the Life Story

We recommend the following ingredients to create a comprehensive Life Story. They are listed here in chronological order, but the events are not necessarily limited to those years. For example, someone may have been in military service throughout her working life.

Childhood

Birthday and birthplace (and/or adoption)
Parents and grandparents
Brothers and sisters
Early education
Pets

Adolescence

Name of high school

Favorite classes

Friends and interests

Hobbies and sports

First job

Young Adulthood

College and work

Marriage(s)/relationship(s)

Family

Clubs and/or community involvement

First home

Military service

Middle Age

Grandchildren

Hobbies

Work/family role

Clubs and organizations

Community involvement

Later years

Life achievements and accomplishments

Hobbies

Travel

Family

Other major ingredients

Ethnicity

Religious background

Awards

Special skills

- Try starting with education. Did your mother graduate from college? She might have been the first one in the family to obtain a college degree, often a source of great pride. Did she go away to college and live in a dorm or stay in her hometown?
- Discover other life events associated with school. Maybe your mother was on the cheerleading squad or winner of the spelling bee. Experiences such as high school proms are memorable and often are photographed for scrapbooks, which can be retrieved and utilized as part of the Life Story.
- Ask about transportation. Early modes of transportation evoke special memories. How did your mother get to school—by bus, by car, or by foot? What was her first car? One California day center director told the authors that a discussion of "my first car" was one of the center's most successful programs. Even participants with poor memory seemed to be able to recall the make and color of their first car and that car's first flat tire. One day, a center participant recalled his car's rumble seat, which drew blank stares from several younger members of the staff. "Does that have something to do with earthquakes?" one aide asked.
- Discuss her first job. Jobs are often the most important way people define themselves. It can be interesting to ask what the person's first wage was. Many young people would certainly be surprised to hear that a wage of less than twenty dollars a week was not uncommon!
- Ask your mother if she can remember her first kiss. This question almost always evokes a laugh, a smile, or a blush.

Young Adulthood

Education, work, and family life often dominate the young adult years. List your knowledge of your mother's marriage and note children. This information can be added to the family tree begun earlier. Are there nieces or nephews or special cousins who made up the extended family?

- Incorporate your mother's higher education (if any) and describe early work or career choices. Many individuals seek higher education during this period or begin working.
- Don't forget wedding details. A wedding can be a highlight of this time of life, and a Life Story should include information about the wedding ceremony, especially any funny stories, such as the groom misplacing the ring or a multilevel cake that collapsed. Wedding pictures, part of most families' archives, can be a marvelous source of family history.
- Obtain as much information as you can about your mother's job or career. Was she a nurse, homemaker, artist, or, like Mary Edith, a pilot? Note any collections or materials from her work that might still be available. A homemaker might have kept an elaborate card file of recipes. If your mother wore a uniform associated with her occupation, it can provide a fun prop for reminiscence.
- Include pictures of the first house, if possible, in the Life Story or see if the image is available via the Internet. Google Earth and other websites may have a picture of the actual house if you can enter the address into the search engine! (The Internet can also give you lots of trivia to discuss about a person's

home town.) Often, this period is one in which a first home was purchased, an act that has enormous symbolic value. Your mother may still remember the amount of their first monthly mortgage payment.

Middle Age

Writing a complete Life Story of a person's middle-age period could fill several books, but again you want to at least highlight major themes. Middle age is a period in life when your mother may have reached the peak of her career. What was her last job before retirement, and were there any noteworthy achievements? It can be important to understand whether your mother's identity is tied to her job. Did she primarily identify herself through her professional world or through her family life, or both?

- Note what hobbies your mother had or what recreational activities she enjoyed. Avocations often develop during this time. Golfers often have spent countless hours thinking, talking, and sometimes anguishing over their game. If your mother was a golfer (or still golfs), did she ever hit a hole in one or win a tournament? Was your mother in a sorority or service club?
- Include an update on the family. Did children marry? Were there grandchildren? Were there family reunions?

Later Years

For many people, retirement provides a chance to pursue a hobby or activity more avidly; the individual who played bridge only once a month can now play three times a week. Another can go salmon fishing every other day during the season. For many people, gardening is a pleasurable activity, and the Life Story should note their favorite flowers and whether they had special success with vegetables. Perhaps one year there was an eighty-pound pumpkin in the garden!

- Record whether your mother had an active retirement period. Former President Jimmy Carter's mother, Miss Lillian, joined the Peace Corps at age sixty-eight. What a mistake it would have been for a biographer to leave out this fact when describing her life!
- Did your mother remain physically active? Some older adults work out at health clubs, bike across the country, or take weekly organized hiking trips. If she decided to spend the retirement years sitting on the front porch watching the world go by, a note can be made to tease her about the rocking chair that occupied her day.
- Was there one "dream-of-a-lifetime" trip or a yearly vacation spot? A special vacation can still be a vivid memory even in a person with dementia. What was the special attraction—a tropical island or a desert hideaway? Are pictures or souvenirs available that can be used for the Life Story?
- Note any volunteer jobs your mother had in a hospital auxiliary, for a local nonprofit organization, or for a church or youth group.
- Record if your mother was a reader, learned any new skills during this time, or developed a new business. Some retired people use this period to enrich their lives through continuing education—formal or informal.

Other Major Ingredients

- Look at your mother's cultural, religious, and ethnic background and what role this background played in her life. Is she Jewish; did she keep kosher? Is English a second language, or does your mother only speak her native language? Were there family traditions celebrating her African-American heritage? Did your mother's grandfather move to California when it was still part of Mexico? Conversely, note if she has no strong religious background. Perhaps she would feel uncomfortable singing gospel songs.
- Record your mother's awards or major achievements. Winning a prize or award is such a major event to individuals that it remains in the memory longer than many other events. Therefore, you should note if your mother was honored as Volunteer or Teacher of the Year or given other awards.
- Ask your mother and other family members if they can recall any other things they feel are important to include in the Life Story. Did she have any strong likes or dislikes? At a day center group, the authors discovered that one participant had answered that question, "Republicans," and another in the same group replied, "Democrats." We tried to steer clear of politics that day.
- Know special phrases she often used. Some people have their own special "trademark" phrases such as "You bet!" or "Two heads are better than one." These can add flavor to your mother's Life Story.
- Don't overlook favorite foods. Many people spend a lot of time thinking about food. Some pride themselves on knowing special recipes or on knowing how to cook foods reflecting their

ethnicity. Food can still be a source of much enjoyment and sensory pleasure for the person.

- Write down your mother's favorite song or type of music. It is important to let people listen to music they enjoy, whether it is Bach, Benny Goodman, or the Beatles.
- Think about what your mother's favorite color is. Often, late into dementia a person can still respond to questions about color and is pleased to be surrounded by items or wear clothing of a favored color.
- Note if your mother enjoys socializing more with women or men. A person will sometimes favor the company of one gender over another. Did your mother have mostly female or male friends?
- Include your mother's special skills. For example, a person will often retain the ability to play a beautiful old song that he or she has played for many years, despite the fact that Alzheimer's disease prevents him or her from learning a simple new song. Other common skills include cooking, sewing, painting, and making crafts.
- Describe the overall personality of your mother before developing dementia. Learning this information is important because old personality patterns often are retained. Was she generally optimistic or pessimistic? What was her problem-solving approach? How was stress handled?
- Update the Life Story regularly! Have there been any major family developments, such as weddings, reunions, or new grandchildren? Has your mother gone on a trip? Has the family given her a new pet?

- Take special note of any successes or happy memories that can be used to benefit the person. You did this in the childhood section, and you should do it throughout. The Life Story should also offer warnings against any painful subjects, phobias, or important information to be avoided.
- Take note if there is "one special thing" that helps define the person, is of special importance, or might be how a person sums up his or her life. Perhaps the person had a lifelong interest in animals, worked as a medical researcher, loved her role as a mother and grandmother, found meaning through her relationship with God or a higher power or her membership in a faith community, or was proud of her lifelong optimism.

Questions That Enrich a Written Life Story

Looking beneath the surface can pay many dividends. Unusual questions can reveal much about the person's attitudes about life. The questions can be asked of friends and family or directly of the person, when possible. The goal is to get an idea of the person's values before the onset of dementia, so questions are written in the past tense, but whenever possible, obtain present-day answers as well.

1. How would the person have enjoyed spending New Year's Eve? It can be revealing to know if he or she would have been in the middle of Times Square, out dancing, or home with a book.
2. Did the person have a favorite book? Would she have preferred a good mystery novel, Shakespeare, the Bible, poetry, an auto repair manual, or *The Farmer's Almanac*?

3. If the person were stuck on a desert island, what three things would he or she wish to have along? (Assume there is food, drink, and shelter.)
4. How would the person's desk have been organized? (If the person did not have a desk, substitute kitchen shelves and drawers, tool box, or barn.)
5. Would the person have looked at life thinking the glass is half-full or half-empty?
6. Would the person have held onto the first dollar he or she made or spent it immediately?

HOW TO USE THE LIFE STORY

Creating the Life Story is one art; using it is another. Here are some key areas where the story helps.

Greeting the Person and Improving Recognition

Depending on the severity of the dementia, the person may or may not recognize a familiar family member, friend, paid in-home worker, or program staff member. Without recognition, the opening moments of any interaction can be difficult or embarrassing if the person cannot remember a face or name. When you use the Life Story, recognition is enhanced. At the Best Friends Day Center, for instance, a care partner said, "Hi there, Harry. You are from one of my favorite cities in the world—New Orleans. What did you like best about living in New Orleans?"

Facts from the Life Story put the person immediately at ease. Sadly, sometimes a family member must even say, "Hello, Mom, it's your son Tony." As hard as this is to do, it is an act of kindness to put the person at ease and compensate for some of the losses of dementia.

Introducing the Person to Others

Introductions serve two primary purposes. First, they build self-esteem and evoke smiles, sometimes putting the person at ease in uncomfortable social situations. Second, the person is introduced to others as a valued member of society, someone good to know. Many long-term care programs debate about whether to address someone by a proper name, such as Mr. Johnson, or by a first name. Although the authors believe that the person with dementia is best addressed by a first name (because it is retained in memory longer), the Life Story will give important information about this subject. If someone is from the South, where society is more formal than in southern California, for example, it is possible that he or she would prefer to be introduced in a more formal fashion, such as "Mr." or "Mrs." Introductions can also be tied to a profession such as "Judge" or "Doctor." Recognizing one's own name is often one of the last cognitive skills lost to Alzheimer's disease. Use the person's preferred name often, be it a proper name or a name defining a relationship ("Dad" or "Sis").

> *I'd like for you to meet my friend, Edith Hayes. She and I have been friends for more years than we both like to admit. Right, Edith? She's a nurse, a master gardener, a mother, a grandmother, and a great-grandmother.*

This technique of introductions is also one that artful activities staff practice in long-term care settings, introducing residents or adult day participants to one another throughout an activity or occasionally during the day.

Reminiscing

Perhaps the most obvious benefit to having a good, comprehensive biography of the person is to allow for reminiscing. We all enjoy sharing memories and old stories and may be able to tell an old story with great detail, and of course, usually with a number of embellishments (think of the classic fish stories).

An Easy Start

If you are overwhelmed by the idea of creating a full Life Story, try this Bullet Card innovation by Dee Carlson, an Alzheimer's care consultant: Take a 5 x 7 card and write down key things a paid worker or visiting family member or friend would need to know about the person. What name should be used to address the person, e.g., Bob or Major Smith? Where was he or she born? Any particular likes or dislikes? How does he or she take coffee in the morning? All of these facts can help someone better relate to, and thus care for, a person with dementia.

Life Story "Bullet Card"

James R. Smith **Age: _____**

Likes to be called J. R.

- Likes his coffee before he gets dressed; little cream, one sugar
- Is very private while bathing; keep a towel around him
- Hates lima beans, okra, and spinach
- Enjoys baseball games
- Tends to pace when upset or angry
- Loves to hear jokes and can tell a few

Persons with Alzheimer's disease still enjoy reminiscing. When looking at an old family photograph, the person may, with cueing, be able to recall some names and relationships. If not, the photograph can still be used to talk about fashions from that era ("Mom, look at the hats ladies used to wear!") or to discuss other interesting items in the photograph ("Mom, is that lady really wearing a foxtail fur piece?"). Memories and impressions of parents and grandparents often remain vivid.

Mary Burmaster loved to be reminded that her grandfather was a beloved country doctor. Staff members at her day center remind her about her grandfather and then they reminisce together, not so much about the details of her grandfather's life but about country doctors in general. They talk about doctors delivering babies, their black bags, and their wish that physicians still made house calls. Whenever possible, staff members incorporate details they know about her grandfather. "Mary, I remember you telling me that his first house call was way back at the turn of the century!"

Early childhood stories, particularly ones involving childhood mischief, are enjoyable to the person. Gently teasing a retired college professor about how he used to skip school can bring laughter. Or someone can be reminded of the time he took his uncle's wool hat and stuck it up the chimney to hide it, only to be found out when a fire was lit and the room filled with smoke!

Margaret Brubaker enjoyed being reminded (and teased) about the times she would play the game of craps. She even taught her son, Jim, how to play. Because she always greeted visitors in such a proper manner and appeared to be very traditional, it was fun to reminisce with her about this hidden and unexpected talent.

Improving Communication Through Clues and Cues

Knowing the Life Story can improve communication because it may provide clues to what the person is saying. For example, if someone with dementia says, "I need to get home, the children, it's getting late," a daughter who is familiar with the person's Life Story might recall that she was a homemaker who made a big dinner for her family every night. The care partner might make a guess and say, "Oh, Mom, don't worry. I have already made a delicious dinner for us. Tonight you get to be spoiled."

The Life Story also helps provide clues, when needed, to allow the person to finish a sentence. If your mother says, "I need to call my husband . . ." and is struggling to find his name, you can supply the name by saying, "You mean your husband, Mike?" If she keeps talking about her childhood but seems unable to supply many details, you can use your knowledge of her Life Story to inquire, "Mom, it must have been wonderful growing up in the pretty town of Walla Walla. Aren't you lucky to have grown up surrounded by those beautiful wheat fields and famous sweet onions?"

Evelyn Talbott had an intense desire to converse. She lit up whenever someone would prompt her about her work, her love of dogs, her interest in dancing, and her enjoyable nature walks. She would use her hands to gesture toward her body, saying with her hands, "Give me more, keep going." People who knew elements of her Life Story found it easy to converse with her, but someone who did not know much about her would find the conversation ended quickly.

Evelyn needed others to do most of the work, to "carry the ball" in conversations.

Designing Appropriate Activities

The Life Story provides many important clues to activities that may have the greatest chance of capturing the person's interest and evoking a positive, joyful response. We can look to the person's Life Story for clues about his or her skills. For example, an accountant diagnosed with Alzheimer's disease certainly will no longer be able to handle a complex transaction, but he or she might enjoy "helping" to add a row of figures. A retired librarian could help organize a collection of magazine clippings and photographs. A former homemaker may enjoy helping to prepare a batch of cookies or folding laundry. A retired shoe salesperson may enjoy looking at wholesale shoe catalogs and "placing" a new order. The possibilities are endless.

Gladys Bell continues her love of quilting as a participant in an adult day program. With a volunteer she enjoys selecting material, deciding on colors that would go well together, cutting quilt pieces, and stitching them together. Others with an interest in quilting join in, and an old-fashioned "quilting bee" becomes a regular event on Gladys's day in the program.

When Gladys takes home the quilt she is working on, the family can enjoy talking about this project, as well as all the articles she has made for the family over the years. This type of activity, common in many day centers, also lends itself to a good home activity. Even children can participate, as well as friends and neighbors.

The Life Story provides a rich source of ideas for "show and tell." If the person created crafts, collected stamps, painted, won bowling trophies, and so forth, the Life Story can note these items, which can then be used one-to-one to reminisce. In one day center, a collection of old neckties can fill an afternoon with discussion and laughter about the varying styles, colors, and widths that came into, out of, and back into fashion.

Tip for Success

If the person believes things about his or her life that are not factually correct, they should be noted in the life story anyway. Don't overemphasize these inaccuracies, but if some of this information is real to the person, you should be prepared to be more accepting and flexible with the "facts." For example, if an attorney who always loved politics now claims he was in the state senate (and he was not), we don't have an issue with addressing him as "Senator" if that gives him pleasure.

Pointing Out Past Accomplishments

One way to honor individuals with dementia is by remembering their accomplishments, and the Life Story helps you point these out. For example, almost all parents like hearing good things about their children. We can point out when someone's grandson is a Little League champion or congratulate the person if his or her daughter has just received a big promotion.

During his four years at Syracuse University, Jack Cooper was a member of the rowing team. He enjoyed being reminded of his important position as the coxswain. As the coxswain, he sat at the end facing the rowers and gave the signal that synchronized the rowers and guided the racing shell. What a thrill to lead the team to victory!

Jack enjoyed being reminded of this accomplishment, and it's a reminder that a care partner can use over and over again! If your friend or family member with dementia has one particularly special accomplishment, make note of it and refer to it often.

Helping to Prevent Challenging Behaviors

Many challenging behaviors are caused by identifiable triggers, such as being overexposed to grandchildren who are too loud, being asked inappropriate questions, or being rushed. However, sometimes behaviors are hard to explain and may stem from more deep-rooted concerns that might only be apparent from the person's Life Story.

Sometimes a behavior can be triggered when sad memories are inadvertently raised. For example, if a person lost family members in a boating accident, there may be problems if a visitor shows photographs of his or her new boat. The person may not be able to explain his or her feelings, but instead might act out or become despondent. In that case, without a good Life Story, it is almost impossible to determine why the nautical discussions are making someone unhappy.

Brevard Crihfield was used to being the boss at work. He enjoyed the sing-along sessions at the day center until one week, when he became angry during the session. The song leader that day had a wonderful voice and was charismatic as he stood in front of the group. However, he was also somewhat directive, and "Crihf" read that as someone standing in front of him, telling him what to do.

When the song leader sat in a chair by the piano to lead the songs instead of standing, Crihf's outbursts stopped. A simple intervention led to a big payoff because Crihf was calmed and the program could go on.

Incorporating Past Daily Rituals

Some individuals have rituals in their daily life, whether it is going to Mass each morning, taking a daily walk, or having a chocolate malt every day at 2 PM. Daily rituals can be utilized in dementia care.

If a person enjoyed a morning newspaper and cup of coffee, let him or her start the day that way. Even when he or she may not be able to fully read a paper or retain the content, there is enormous symbolic value in simply holding it and turning the pages. Reading a newspaper suggests to others that one is educated, informed, and interested in the world. Offering the person a cup of coffee is a social interaction as well as a gift, and the coffee's warmth and aroma may stimulate positive thoughts. One family told us that when they discovered these rituals, their father stayed busy and satisfied for more than an hour every morning.

Nancy Zechman loved nothing better than a long daily drive in the country. Often, Nancy climbed into her husband Fred's blue truck well before the scheduled time of 4 PM, saying, "Let's go, Fred."

Driving into the country was an activity that both Nancy and Fred enjoyed; it also relieved the anxiety that sometimes began to build up for Nancy late in the day as she grew tired.

Celebrating Family Traditions

It can be helpful to know of family traditions, including ways that a family celebrated Christmas or the religious holidays, how someone celebrated family birthdays or New Year's Eve, or if they had traditions around special events such as the birth of a new baby.

> *Alison Tobin, Assisted Living Manager at Piedmont Gardens in Oakland, surveyed residents and family members in their memory care community called The Grove about holiday traditions. During December, the staff made note of and celebrated each resident's traditions, including special foods such as mincemeat pies, favorite holiday movies like the Jimmy Stewart classic* It's a Wonderful Life, *and favorite holiday songs. Alison explains that one resident had a tradition of making handmade Christmas ornaments as gifts. She lit up with joy when reminded of this tradition, and so staff helped her create new ornaments as gifts for her family.*

Traditions and rituals stay with us in our memories. Touching on them can promote feelings of comfort and happiness.

Broadening the Caregiving Network and Resources

A Life Story can remind families, agencies, adult day center directors, and residential care facility operators of the richness of the person's past. In many cases, the person volunteered in a faith community group or in civic and social clubs. In some cases, a person belonged to a special military unit, the police or fire department, or a trade union.

From the Life Story, a list can be made of potential organizations or volunteers who can provide help to the family or volunteer support to the service program. The local fire department could let a retired firefighter have a ride in an off-duty truck or a church group could arrange a rotation of weekly social visits.

Because the day center staff knew that Nancy Zechman was an avid tennis player, they looked to her social contacts and friends for potential volunteer help. Her tennis partners at the Lexington Tennis Club were contacted, and Nancy's close friend, Jody Bollum, agreed to be with Nancy at the day center once a week. When together, Jody helped Nancy feel safe and secure, in part because they had many stories and experiences in common.

Don't be afraid to ask for help from groups that your family member has supported. Many individuals and groups want to help and only need suggestions about how.

LIFE STORY OF REBECCA MATHENY RILEY

Rebecca's family compiled her Life Story, which proved helpful later when she became a participant in the Best Friends Day Center, and still later when she was admitted to the Christian Health Center, a nursing home in Lexington, Kentucky. Here, in italics, we explore how such a story can be used—what care partners can talk about, watch out for, celebrate, and so on—in everyday care. Use this as a model to create a life story for your friend or family member.

Rebecca is the oldest child *[talk about responsibility of first-born]*, born January 8, 1925, to Elsie Arnold and S. F. Matheny. She is the first granddaughter on both sides of her family *[unique family story]*. Rebecca and her only sister, Mary Frances, eighteen months younger, were very close as children and remain intimate friends *[likes talking about childhood stories]*. When Rebecca was only three years old, her mother died *[source of sadness]* and her grandparents became parents to Rebecca and her little sister.

Rebecca adored her grandparents and named them Grandpa and Grandma *[talk about names used to describe grandparents]*. Her grandmother came to this country in 1892 from Austria, and some family members still reside there *[discuss traditions]*.

The little girls were happy-go-lucky as they played in the creek that ran through their grandparents' farm. Catching frogs and tadpoles that lived in the creek was a favorite pastime on a hot summer day. On autumn days, they enjoyed gathering hickory nuts and walnuts that had fallen from the many trees on the farm *[reminisce about gathering nuts, talk about the tastes and uses of nuts]*.

Grandpa had lots of animals, including one horse that he allowed the little girls to ride alone. This horse was very slow and deliberate and always dependable as he carried the girls safely on his back. One day this trusty horse became frightened and, as he ran faster and faster, the girls "held on for dear life." Rebecca remembers the scary ride and how happy they were when a neighbor rescued them *[memorable story that made a big impact; can be repeated]*.

Rebecca had many friends at school *[create a collage of school-related pictures]*. A favorite game to play with her classmates was the game of hide-and-seek *[Rebecca enjoys games—perhaps try charades]*. When Rebecca was in the first grade, she invited her entire class to come home with her after school *[tease her about this]*. This was a big surprise to Grandpa and Grandma. Although they all had a great time playing at the farm, she remembers a serious discussion about asking permission before inviting so many friends to visit *[discussion about discipline then and now]*.

Rebecca and Mary Frances were often responsible for doing the dishes after supper to help their grandmother. They argued about whose turn it was to clean up the kitchen *[reminisce about chores]*.

As Rebecca grew older, she wondered about her mother: "What was she really like?" "Why did she have to leave me when I was such a little girl?" Her father remarried and she now had two brothers, Sam and Earl. Although Grandma and Grandpa were wonderful "parents," Rebecca often had sad thoughts about not knowing her mother *[remember this if she expresses feelings of sadness; could be old memories*].

Even as a young girl, Rebecca was goal oriented. She had a determined spirit and a mind of her own, refusing to take "no" for an answer *[speak in positives instead of in negatives]*. That spirit remains very much a part of her. She always wanted to be helpful and productive, especially to others in great need. She was motivated to learn, making her an excellent student *[some key personality traits—motivated, goal oriented, helpful]*.

During her youth, Rebecca was a member of the Methodist church and active in the Epworth League sponsored by the church. Her religious faith fed her spirit and desire to be helpful. She often made known her life goals: to be a nurse, serve as a missionary, and marry a minister *[religion is very important to her]*.

During her years at Stanford High School, Rebecca played in the band *[check to see if she still plays any instruments]*. She was also a member of the Girl's Reserve Club and graduated with honors *[opportunity for congratulations]*. After graduation, she enrolled in nurse's training at Good Samaritan Hospital in Lexington, Kentucky. As a nursing student *[likes to be reminded she is a nurse, complimented on past achievements as a nurse]*, she met her husband while he was a patient in the hospital *[funny story about how they met]*. Although nursing students at that time were not allowed to remain in school after marriage, Rebecca relied on her determined spirit *[note determination]* and became the first married nursing student at the hospital *[note as major accomplishment]*.

On April 20, 1945, she married Jo M. Riley, an ordained minister in the Christian Church (Disciples of Christ) *[talk about wedding traditions]*. His pastorates took them to Kokomo, Indiana; Wilson, North Carolina; Decatur, Illinois; Louisville, Kentucky; and Centralia, Illinois. She taught church classes for children and young adults and was very supportive of all church activities. She served on a national Week of Compassion committee for her church *[compliment her on leadership ability]*. This was a special honor for Rebecca, giving her the opportunity to use her expertise on a national level *[this was a happy time for her]*.

Rebecca was nominated Mother of the Year while living in Kokomo, Indiana, and was President of the Minister's Wives Organization of Illinois. These honors are very special to her. The community also benefited from Rebecca's helping hands. She was a Girl Scout leader for several years *[praise her for her contributions to the community]*.

Rebecca and Jo became parents of three children: Lucinda, Joetta, and Louis *[use the names for conversational cues]*. Lucinda and her son, Josh, live in Washington, D.C. Joetta is married to William Parris and lives in North Carolina. Louis and his wife, Joy, have three children, Ian, Tristan, and Grant; they live in Tennessee. Rebecca has always been family oriented; her family comes first *[any mention of her family always makes her feel special and proud]*.

Rebecca and Jo owned a cottage on Crystal Lake in Michigan. Each summer the family vacationed there *[could be the source of old photos or mementos, fun memories]*. Given an hour's notice, Rebecca said they could be packed up and ready to go. This was a wonderful place for the children to play *[talk about her children's experiences each summer at the lake]*. The cottage was located just a stone's throw from the water. Swimming and enjoying their rowboat were great ways for the family to spend time together. Also, family and friends returned each year to nearby cottages. Often, these friends gathered with the Riley family for picnics at special locations on the lake. One of Rebecca's favorite activities was a breakfast picnic on a hot summer day. The sand dunes nearby were very tall and inviting to climb after the picnic *[tease her that she couldn't wait to be the first one up the hill]*.

Cooking is an art for Rebecca. Wherever she lived, she learned how to prepare local dishes and delighted in serving these dishes to visitors to the community. Two of Rebecca's specialties were "popcorn" cake and persimmon pudding *[she may enjoy being asked her opinion about recipes, tasting unusual dishes]*. Rebecca remembers preparing a reception for 500 people—what a big task!

In 1972 Rebecca returned to school to earn a bachelor's of science degree in nursing, and in 1974 she received a master's degree in education from Spaulding College. She taught nursing students until she was diagnosed with Alzheimer's disease in July 1984. Spaulding College, Jefferson Community College, and Centralia College all benefited from her gift of teaching *[likes to do things that evoke skills of teaching]*.

After their children were grown, Jo and Rebecca traveled to England, Scotland, Australia, New Zealand, Israel, Jordan, China, Russia, Austria, and other European countries. While in Austria, they visited Rebecca's grandmother's home, the fulfillment of a dream for Rebecca *[pictures, mementos?]*.

Rebecca also enjoys classical music, knitting, sewing, reading, and homemaking. Her favorite hymn is "Amazing Grace." Her dog, Corky, is a constant companion, especially since the diagnosis of Alzheimer's disease. Corky reminds her of her childhood pet dog, Briar *[all good activity ideas]*.

When Rebecca was diagnosed with Alzheimer's disease she shared her feelings about the result openly and honestly as long as she was able to do so. Rebecca wanted to do everything she could to be of help to others.

Authors' note: Woven through all her roles in life is a common thread: Rebecca was always a teacher. She probably did her best teaching after she was diagnosed with Alzheimer's disease. Rebecca was determined to make a difference. She enrolled in research studies to help find the cause of the disease, and she taught everyone who would listen what it is like to live in the world of Alzheimer's disease.

Rebecca died in August of 1999. At her memorial service, it was noted that "she lives on in the lives of her many students around the world." She lives on as well as a symbol of strength and courage through this book.

The life story can be supplemented with photographs of the person. At right, Rebecca is pictured from her childhood (seen here with her younger sister, Mary Frances), through her early nursing career, her marriage to Jo, and her young adulthood, raising a family.

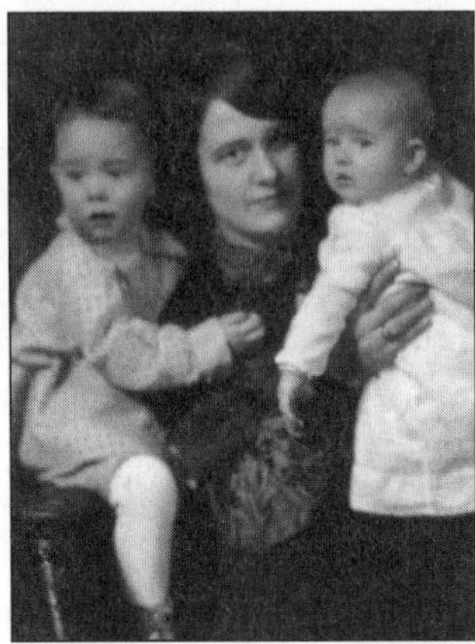

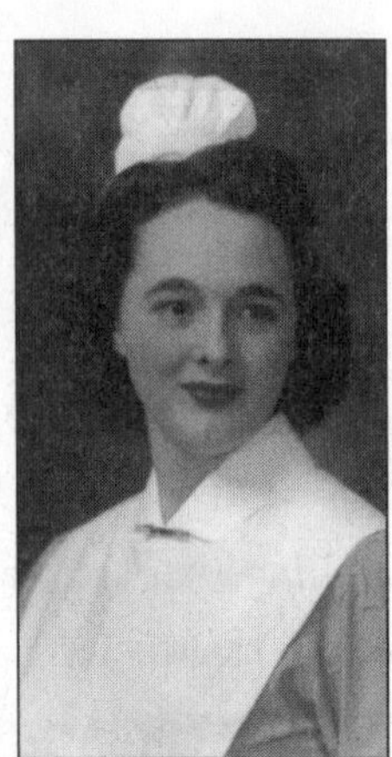

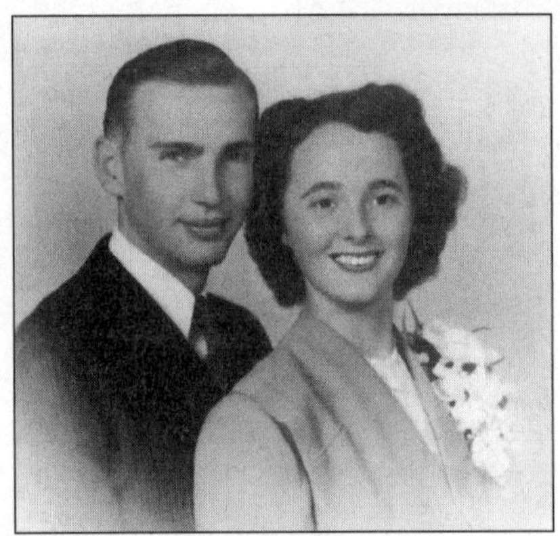

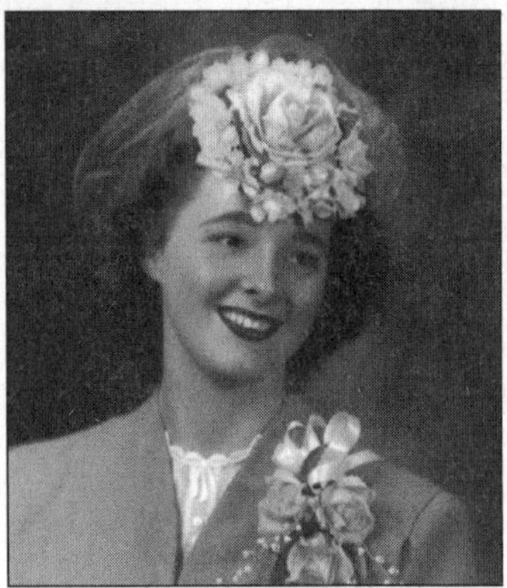

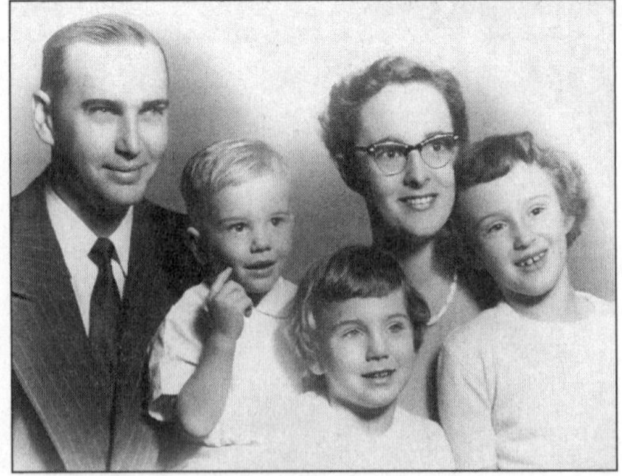

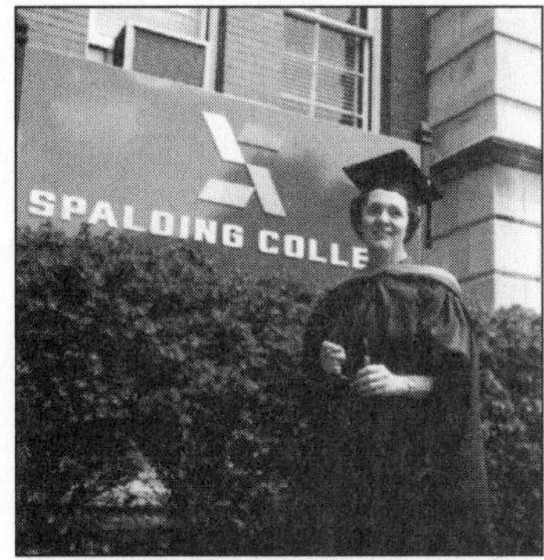

Rebecca graduated with a bachelor's of science in nursing. As her dementia progressed, she found comfort in playing with her dogs and traveling with Jo. Even when she required continuous care at a facility, she still had her soft eyes and warm smile.

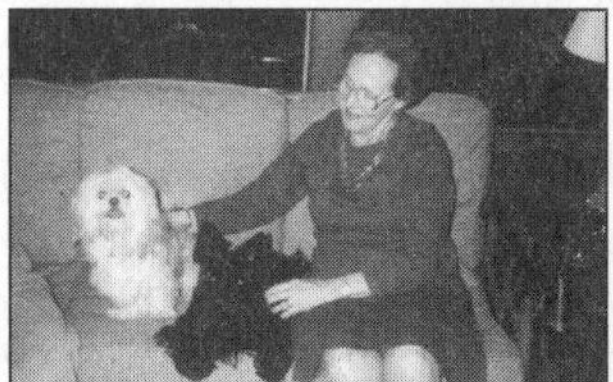

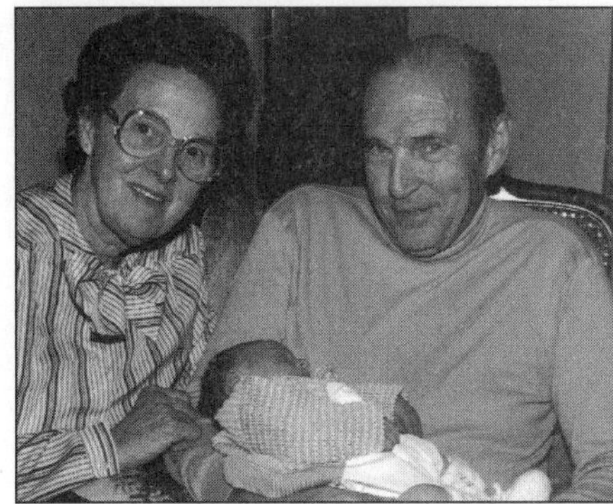

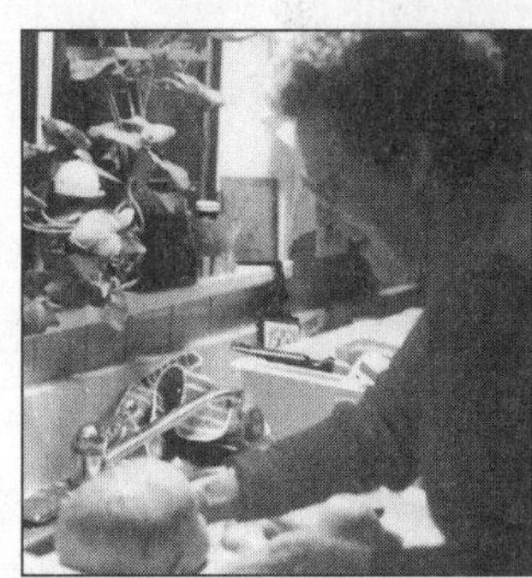

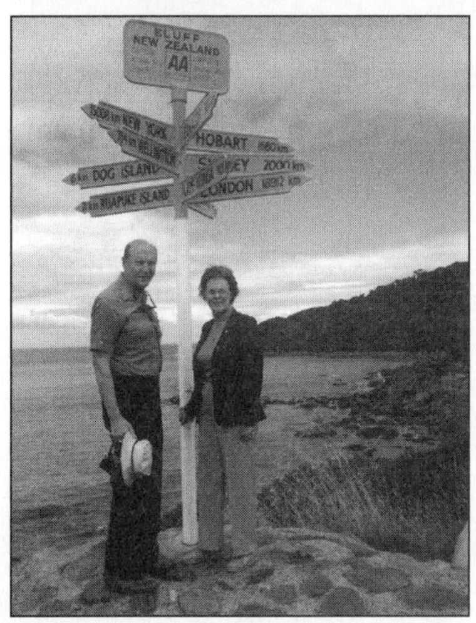

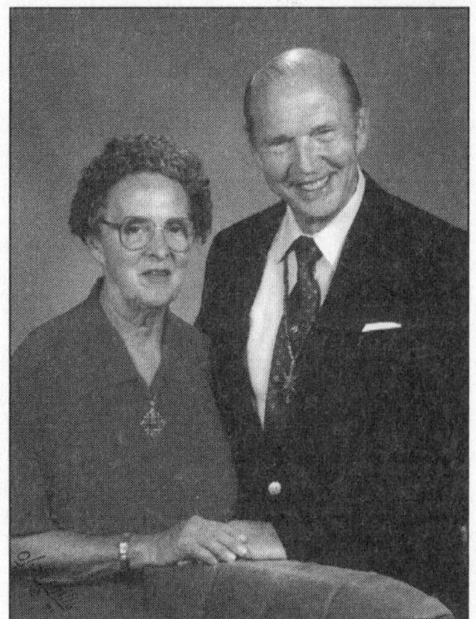

CONCLUSION

William M. Small Jr., president and owner of the Fountainview Center, a dementia-specific residential care center in Atlanta, told us that he and his staff would read obituaries of residents who died and learn new and surprising facts about their lives. Mr. Small said that after a period of time he became angry and frustrated by the fact that he and his staff did not know the residents as well as he felt they should. The staff vowed to work with families to enhance and expand the life stories of their residents.

Today he feels that quality of care has improved immensely. "We now read the obituaries with love, affection, and sadness for the loss but with no surprises about the person's past." The families also appreciate very much that an activities staff member knows Mother's nickname, that the certified nursing assistant asks about a child by name, that the nurse comments on the beautiful weavings made by the resident and hanging in her room, or that the receptionist can comment on a past achievement as the resident walks by.

These are all small moments of connection for both the person with dementia and the staff at the Fountainview Center. They do not cost any money, are not subject to regulations, and do not require advanced training. They only require staff taking a moment to be a Best Friend to the resident in their care.

Best Friends Pointers

- During your daily interaction with a friend or family member with dementia, pick a favorite subject from his or her Life Story to discuss. You can also use items around the house or apartment for reminiscence, such as a family photo album, bowling trophy, or military medal.
- Creating a written Life Story and sharing it with anyone involved in the person's care is an essential step for providing outstanding care.
- In collecting the Life Story, involve the person whenever possible; ask friends and family to contribute as well.
- If a full-blown Life Story feels overwhelming, start by creating a quick list of the top ten things to know about the person on a 5 x 7 index card.
- Use Internet tools to further research the Life Story and to view images from the person's hometown or past.

6

THE "KNACK"

Basic Principles of Dementia Care

In families, residential care programs, adult day centers, and in-home care situations around the world, you find people who stand out, who seem to have a "magic touch" in their work with, or care of, persons with Alzheimer's disease and other dementia. These situations include:

- The beloved nursing assistant who can rise to any occasion and always seems to say or do the right thing.
- The adult son who does things he never dreamed he could and now helps his mother with personal care, including bathing and dressing.
- The husband who gives loving care to his wife, uses local services, and approaches his tasks in a joyful way, seemingly avoiding the burnout that affects so many care partners.

- The nursing home activities director who is always coming up with ideas for a consistently rich and innovative activity program.
- The in-home worker who knocks on the door, smiles, gives the person with dementia a hug, and builds a great relationship with the person he or she is helping.

What is the difference between care partners who struggle and care partners who succeed? Some of us have more financial resources to draw on, which can make a positive difference. A large and supportive family can help. In professional settings, a liberal budget and successful volunteer program can enrich programs. Yet some care partners and some institutions with almost unlimited resources still struggle, while others with limited resources thrive.

The individuals and institutions who succeed have mastered the "knack" of caregiving. We define "knack" as the art of doing difficult things with ease or clever tricks or strategies. Some individuals are simply born with knack; their personality and sensibility help them to be wonderful care partners. Cynthia Lilly, National Memory Care and Dementia Program Director for Atria Senior Living, has the knack:

> *I always make the most of my first five minutes with a person with dementia, particularly if I'm trying to encourage them to do something like come to lunch or attend an exercise class. I find that when I greet them by name, approach them with a smile or hug, use their Life Story, and try to really be present for them, everything goes better. The "no" becomes a "yes." Sometimes these five minutes save thirty minutes; sometimes it saves the whole day!*

Families struggling with a person who has behaviors that are challenging will do well to remember Cynthia's five-minute strategy. Getting off to a positive start fosters cooperation and can help you get a task like dressing or bathing accomplished.

Even if you are not sure if you have the knack, anyone can improve their dementia caregiving by understanding some basic ingredients and how they are used.

THE INGREDIENTS OF KNACK

The knack of caring for a person with dementia comes from possessing many skills and abilities—ones that will come to you once you see how they work and have the chance to practice them. The following are the elements of knack that are central to the Best Friends approach.

Being Well-Informed

Care partners with knack learn as much as they can about dementia in order to be better informed of new research and treatments, to learn caregiving tips, and to locate new community resources. They attend conferences and workshops, study reputable websites, subscribe to appropriate newsletters, and talk to other families coping with dementia. They recognize that the more one knows about dementia, the less stressful the difficult job of caregiving becomes.

Having Empathy

Care partners with knack have taken time to imagine what it would be like to have dementia. This helps friends and families understand the world of the person in their care and how that world can be difficult and frightening. Empathy also teaches that many of the person's odd or upsetting behaviors are caused by their attempts to make sense of their world—a world clouded by dementia.

Respecting the Basic Rights of the Person

Care partners with knack regard persons with dementia as individuals who deserve loving, high-quality care. They give persons as much say in their care as possible and try to keep them productive in work and play as long as is realistic. They use the Alzheimer's Disease Bill of Rights (see page 55) as their touchstone.

Maintaining Integrity

Care partners with knack approach problems and decision making with an attitude of goodwill toward the person, and they approach care in an ethical fashion. When they withhold information or work their way out of problematic situations, they do so out of concern and in the best interests of the person. For example, a care partner who decides not to tell her mother that they are going to visit an adult day center for the first time and "surprises" her mother with the visit may in fact be withholding information, but this decision is made with integrity.

Employing Finesse

Care partners with knack are able to utilize the art of finesse to respond to difficult situations. They use skillful, subtle, tactful, diplomatic, and well-timed maneuvers to handle problems. In the game of bridge, finesse is taking a trick economically. The same holds true in dementia care; as care partners we want to win a few hands. If a person says "I want to go home," and you respond "Soon," you are using finesse to give the person the answer he or she wants to hear. Some family members struggle with this strategy, feeling that they are lying or being deceitful. As long as care partner integrity is maintained, the authors believe that skillful finesse is part of good dementia care.

Elements of Knack

Knack is the art of doing difficult things with ease or clever tricks and strategies. The elements of knack include:

Being well-informed
Having empathy
Respecting the basic rights of the person
Maintaining integrity
Employing finesse
Knowing it is easier to get forgiveness than to get permission
Using common sense
Communicating skillfully
Maintaining optimism
Setting realistic expectations
Using humor
Employing spontaneity
Maintaining patience
Developing flexibility
Staying focused
Being nonjudgmental
Valuing the moment
Maintaining self-confidence
Using cueing tied to the Life Story

Connecting with the spiritual

Taking care of oneself

Planning ahead

Knowing It Is Easier to Get Forgiveness Than to Get Permission

Care partners with knack know that sometimes decisions must be made for the person. They know that asking permission works with a person with intact cognitive abilities but is not always the best option with someone who has dementia. When the person does become angry or upset at the care partner for making a decision (for example, throwing dirty clothes in the laundry or cleaning up a messy house), you may find it expedient to simply "take the blame" or apologize for the "misunderstanding." The person will soon forget the incident, but meanwhile you have been able to take care of a task that needed doing.

Using Common Sense

Care partners with knack exercise common sense. They are not afraid to seek simple solutions to complex problems. Examples of commonsense ideas you can try include: eliminating caffeine when the person has problems sleeping, making extra sets of keys in case a set is hidden or lost, having the person wear an identification bracelet, not making a fuss over things that really don't matter, and making extra photographs of the person to share with others in case he or she wanders away.

Communicating Skillfully

Care partners with knack communicate skillfully, cueing the person with appropriate words from his or her Life Story, using positive body language, and knowing the right and wrong ways to ask and answer questions. Good communication also involves skillful listening, and the best care partners work hard to help the person better communicate. Find out more about communication in Chapter 7.

Maintaining Optimism

Care partners with knack try to look beyond dementia and remember the good things in life. They take joy in even small pleasures that can come from time spent with their loved one with dementia. Care partners maintain a sense of hope that the future will be brighter and that one day a cure for Alzheimer's disease will be found. They try to instill this sense of optimism and hope in the person with the disease.

Setting Realistic Expectations

Expectations that are too high or too low can be frustrating to both care partner and the person. Be realistic. What can the person still do and enjoy? What tasks will lead to success or satisfaction? What might prove frustrating or evoke failure? Achieving this balance is part of the art of knack.

Using Humor

Care partners with knack are not afraid to tell funny stories and jokes, or to laugh when humorous things happen. They understand that even when the person does not "get" a funny story or joke, laughter and good feelings are contagious. The person will absorb these good feelings. Another key element of humor is that care partners should not be afraid to make fun of themselves. Self-deprecation preserves dignity and is a small price to pay to make the person feel better about his or her own circumstances.

Employing Spontaneity

Although persons with dementia do respond to routines, they don't like strict schedules! After all, the schedule is someone else's planning, not theirs. A day of working in the garden planned by the care partner might get interrupted by an hour of unplanned bird watching when colorful cardinals are spotted in the trees. Go with the flow sometimes! It is healthy for the person and for you.

Maintaining Patience

Care partners with knack realize that it takes the person longer to do things and longer to respond to words and events. The act of dressing can take an hour, but it may be an hour during which the person is focused and does not feel lost or lonely. If you do not have an hour to spend helping the person dress, creative solutions can make life run smoother (e.g., use clothes with Velcro fasteners or simplified outfits). All of us occasionally lose our patience, but getting frustrated and angry tends to make matters worse.

Developing Flexibility

It is important to examine oneself and develop greater flexibility as a care partner. Some individuals have lived their lives with great discipline, getting things done on time and adhering to a schedule. This tendency may be helpful in many ways but not if the care partner is rigid or inflexible; persons with dementia want to set their own pace.

Staying Focused

Care partners with knack learn the importance of focus. With all of the distractions around us, it can be hard at times to give the person the attention needed to provide good care. The knack of focus involves really listening to and seeing the person and getting the most out of every interaction. For instance, when helping a person get dressed, turn off the television and take the time to be together and decide together on what colors to wear. Focus also involves putting your own concerns or problems on hold during this time. Anxiety in the care partner, for example, can show up in facial expressions or in vocal tones and can be misread or misunderstood by the person.

Being Nonjudgmental

Care partners with knack work on being nonjudgmental toward the person, family, friends, and themselves. Stress and strain are inherent in caregiving, and they can be increased when friends and family are not always present when needed, or say the wrong thing, or let you down. Of course, it can be very easy to be angry at or disappointed in the person despite the care partner's best intentions. Care partners may not always be at their best either and must learn not to be too hard on themselves.

Valuing the Moment

Care partners with knack know the importance of living in and valuing the moment. A pleasant lunch, time spent arranging flowers, or a fun game of cards may soon be forgotten, but it can be pleasurable for everyone in the moment. This seems particularly important when discussing dementia because affected individuals often lose the past and don't think about the future—the moment is all they have.

Maintaining Self-Confidence

Care partners with knack exhibit self-confidence in their interactions with the person. To be confident, we need to feel that we know what we are doing, have a plan of action, and have some successes to make us feel that we are doing the right thing. Often, this inner strength can be sensed by the person, who may then let go of his or her own concerns or fears. Conversely, if care partners, family members, or professionals are tentative in their actions, the person may sense these feelings and become uneasy.

Using Cueing Tied to the Life Story

Care partners with knack are able to incorporate the Life Story into all aspects of care, cueing the person to remember certain names, places, and things; telling familiar stories; and reminding him or her of past achievements. Even using just a few facts from the person's Life Story can improve the caregiving environment and encourage cooperation.

Connecting with the Spiritual

Care partners with knack fulfill their own spiritual or religious needs and realize that the person also has a need to be loved, appreciated, and known, even though he or she may have to depend upon others to help fulfill these needs. See Chapter 9 for a more extended discussion about the impact of dementia on spirituality and religious practices.

Taking Care of Yourself

Care partners with knack find time for themselves to maintain friendships, exercise, and eat well; they do not let their identity become totally wrapped up in the caregiving role. They attend support groups for emotional support and community connections. They learn more about dementia through conferences and workshops. Look for more information about being your own best friend in Chapter 11.

Planning Ahead

Care partners with knack identify and utilize local services sooner rather than later. Also, care partners with knack have made it a priority to put the person's financial and legal affairs in order. This process should include a contingency plan in case the care partner becomes incapacitated or dies. Who will then care for the person? These are important decisions that should not be neglected by the primary care partner.

LET'S PRACTICE KNACK IN DEMENTIA CARE

Following are some common scenarios that care partners encounter when dealing with individuals with Alzheimer's disease and other dementia. A number of situations are presented comparing dementia care that has "no knack" to that with "knack." Some of the common threads running through all the examples are good listening, empathy, humor, creativity, skilled communication, and lots of patience. Remember, if you have met one person with Alzheimer's disease, you have met only one person with Alzheimer's disease; every individual and every situation is different. Thus, the following examples may or may not be appropriate to all situations. We hope readers will be inspired by these examples of knack, or dementia care at its best, and apply the lessons to their own situations.

Desire to Go Home

A wife is perplexed that her husband wants to go home, even though he is at the house they have lived in for twenty years. She cannot imagine why he feels like a stranger in his own home. He often says, "I want to go home, I want to go home."

No-Knack Approach

"This is your home and has been for twenty years! I can get the deed out of the files to show you. Remember how we worked so hard to pay for this property?"

Caregiving with Knack

"Tell me more about that big red brick house of yours in Milwaukee. Tell me about home."

Why It Works

The no-knack approach demonstrates the futility of trying to win an argument with a person with dementia or explain things in detail. The husband probably picked up the wife's agitated and frustrated tone of voice. He really thinks he is not at home, or he is remembering a different home from his past, or his words might not have literal meaning and be more about a feeling than a place.

The approach with knack allows for the possibility that wanting to go home may mean getting back to where things make sense again. Asking him to say more about it might give him room to talk more about his feelings or describe the home. Perhaps after some discussion he will move on to another topic or be satisfied.

Feelings of Sadness

"I'm very sad today. Nobody loves me anymore," a mother says to her daughter-in-law.

No-Knack Approach

"I don't think it's good to feel sorry for yourself. You've got so much to be thankful for. You've got lots of family, including your granddaughter, Kimiko, in Japan who is visiting you soon, your cousins in Ohio, and your sister in New York. You were happy yesterday; just try to enjoy yourself today."

Caregiving with Knack

"I'm sorry you're feeling blue today. I feel that way now and then too, but you know you are my friend, and I love you a whole bunch. Your granddaughter, Kimiko, will be coming soon. That should be lots of fun."

Why It Works

The no-knack response fails to acknowledge the person's feelings. The daughter-in-law presents too much information to the person all at once. Telling a person, in effect, to "Shape up!" is usually not helpful in any situation where someone is feeling blue.

The approach with knack affirms the person's feelings of loneliness—not judging, just listening and accepting. We don't always need to "cheer up" a person with dementia; sadness is part of life. The daughter-in-law admits having similar feelings, which helps the person believe that she is not alone, that these feelings happen to all of us. Her statement of love is heartwarming and uplifting.

Problems with Bathing

A family is exasperated because their mother struggles with them when it's time for her bath. She insists she has already bathed that day or makes other excuses. When they finally get her in the shower or tub, the bathing process is another struggle.

No-Knack Approach

"Mom, if you don't get into the tub we'll have to put you in a nursing home. You stink! Don't you have any pride anymore?"

Caregiving with Knack

Prepare the bath in advance, and use a calm tone of voice. Use some positive language such as, "It is time to go to the spa," or "Let's clean up before going out to lunch." Ask the doctor to write an "Rx" or "prescription" for bathing. Jump in the shower with Mom or try sponge baths (which can still be effective).

How Are You Doing with Knack?

Rate how you're doing using knack as a caregiver in these different areas:

	Lots of Knack		Knack		No Knack
Am reassuring and supportive	1	2	3	4	5
Try new activities	1	2	3	4	5
Treat the person as an adult	1	2	3	4	5
Am optimistic	1	2	3	4	5
Use positive language	1	2	3	4	5
Am patient and flexible	1	2	3	4	5
Use humor	1	2	3	4	5
Congratulate and compliment	1	2	3	4	5
Don't ask questions that he/she can't answer	1	2	3	4	5
Listen carefully	1	2	3	4	5
Am affectionate, loving	1	2	3	4	5
Use common sense	1	2	3	4	5
Do not argue	1	2	3	4	5
Keep a routine	1	2	3	4	5
Allow person to discuss feelings	1	2	3	4	5
Become familiar with available resources	1	2	3	4	5

After you have worked through this simple exercise, do not despair if you have many scores closer to 5 (No knack) than 1 (Lots of knack). Vow to work on one element each week, and gradually go through the list, making improvements wherever possible.

Why It Works

The no-knack approach fails to understand the fears that a person with memory loss and confusion can have about bathing. The person may associate bathing with being cold, uncomfortable, embarrassed, or out of control. The bullying will only make matters worse. The approach with knack shows preparedness and creativity. Here, the care partner understands that a gentle touch may be best.

Sexual Behavior

One of the most upsetting experiences for a care partner is when the person makes an inappropriate sexual advance. What should happen if a man with dementia makes a sexual advance toward his daughter?

No-Knack Approach

Angry and distressed, the daughter says, "What's wrong with you? Stop that immediately!"

Caregiving with Knack

"Daddy, it's Mary, your daughter. Look what I have here—a photograph of Mother. Isn't she pretty?"

Why It Works

The no-knack approach fails to recognize that the person is most likely confused about identity; daughters often look like their mothers, and he may be remembering himself as a much younger man. If the person thinks his daughter is his wife, his behavior does not seem so out of the ordinary.

The above response with knack is a sensitive one in so many ways. The daughter clearly identifies herself in one sentence by saying, "Daddy, it's Mary, your daughter." Then, by showing her father a picture of her mother, she provides further cueing about roles and identities. Finally, the daughter approaches the situation in a calm, nonjudgmental fashion.

It is also important to note that sometimes the label of sexual inappropriateness is applied incorrectly. If a person begins undressing, it might be because he or she is too warm. A man might unzip his pants to go to the bathroom, not to expose himself.

Angry Outbursts

A mother yells at her son who is visiting her at her assisted living home, "You are late. I've been waiting for you for hours. I am so angry at you!" (The son isn't late. He always visits around dinnertime, but his mother has lost track of time.)

No-Knack Approach

"Mom, I'm not late. I always visit you at dinner. You haven't been waiting for hours and I'm hurt that you'd get angry at me when I always come to visit you."

Caregiving with Knack

"Mom, I'm so sorry. The traffic was terrible. I'll do better next time. I love you!"

Why It Works

The no-knack approach doesn't solve anything and it reminds his mother about her disability. It may make the son feel better in the moment to get his feelings off his chest, but does it help the situation to prove that Mom is wrong and he is right? No.

The approach with knack recognizes that the mother's forgetfulness and confusion created the situation. It is sensitive and understanding for the son to apologize, even when, in fact, he is right and she is wrong!

Repetition

Even when the person has just eaten, he or she may have forgotten or be fixated on food: "When is lunch? When is lunch? Let's eat."

No-Knack Approach

"How many times do I have to tell you that we just had lunch? Please be quiet, you're driving me crazy! You just go on and on and on!"

Caregiving with Knack

"Sis, we'll have a meal soon. Here's a piece of fruit to tide you over."

OR

"Sis, let's put on some of that New Orleans jazz music we love so much and see who can still dance the best. Do you remember our first double date?"

Why It Works

The no-knack approach fails because being reprimanded can make the person defensive, even angry, and does little to end the repetition.

The approach with knack ("We'll have a meal soon") validates her question. The sister's offer to put on old music and her question about their first double date are wonderful distractions that, it is hoped, will break the pattern of repetitive questions.

Dilemmas with Driving

A caregiving family is terribly upset and concerned that Father refuses to give up driving, despite his recent diagnosis of Alzheimer's disease.

No-Knack Approach

"Dad, we followed you around town. You're a terrible driver. You've got Alzheimer's, and you're going to kill someone."

Caregiving with Knack

(Encouraging a doctor to report Dad's condition to the Department of Motor Vehicles [DMV] and then learning that he has failed a written and driving test.) "Dad, I can't believe they've cancelled your license. We'll look into this, but you can't drive without a license! Let's see about retaking that driving test in a few weeks."

Why It Works

The no-knack approach could turn the person against you, will probably not change his desire to drive, and is overly confrontational. Often, the more you push as a care partner, the more the person pushes back! The approach with knack allows someone else to become the bad guy—the doctor, the insurance company, or the DMV. Care partners have also employed other tricks such as disabling the car or lending it to a relative.

CONCLUSION

Even care partners with knack don't get it right all the time. The nature of Alzheimer's disease and other dementia is such that there are always good and bad days (for the person with dementia and for the care partners). An activity or approach may work wonders one day and fail the next. Yet care partners with knack are always willing to try something different and adapt, knowing that approaching problems with knack will never make matters worse. Knack helps you make the best of any situation.

Consider this case of a certified nursing assistant (CNA) at Karrington Cottages in Rochester, Minnesota:

The CNA accompanied a resident with dementia to her room to help her get ready for bed. As they walked to the resident's room, the woman insisted that she wanted to help the CNA get to bed. She said she had to do this before she could go to bed herself. Thinking on her feet, the CNA went to an empty room, slid under the covers of the bed, and allowed the resident to tuck her in for the night. The person then went to her own room, and another staff member helped her get to bed. Here the CNA let the resident recall the comforts of home and a time when she tucked in her own children. It was caregiving with knack.

Best Friends Pointers

- Using elements of the knack are a key part of the Best Friends approach and will help you enjoy more success in navigating the challenges of dementia.
- Don't despair if the knack doesn't come easily for you. Keep working at it and you will develop more knack every day.
- People with knack employ common sense and strive to keep their sense of humor. Trust your instincts, take one day at a time, and try to keep laughter in your life even on those tough days.
- Having the knack of good care is not just about kindness; it provides tools to turn the "no" into a "yes," make personal care easier, and build a more successful relationship with the person.

III

THE BEST FRIENDS APPROACH IN ACTION

7

CONNECTING

Communicating with "Knack"

At a support group meeting, one man expressed frustration that the notes he was leaving on the refrigerator door for his wife with Alzheimer's disease were not working. He had hoped the notes could serve as important reminders whenever he left her alone in their mobile home to run a brief errand. A typical note might be "Take your medicine at noon" or "Don't leave the house!"

He might as well have been leaving the notes in an ancient language. Why? Because his wife might read the notes and not understand them; might read the notes, but then, due to her poor memory, almost immediately forget the message; or might not even remember to read them at all! Refrigerator notes, even with lots of cute magnets drawing attention to them, normally don't work or become ineffective over time.

The loss of communication takes its toll on the relationship between the person and his or her care partner. It makes it much harder to get the person dressed or to discuss everyday problems and concerns. If something wonderful happens—a new grandchild, a successful fund-raiser you have chaired, a published poem in an anthology—you may not be able to fully communicate these experiences to the person with dementia. Husbands and wives may no longer be able to talk over problems and concerns or share in important decisions. Adult children may no longer be able to count on a parent for helpful advice. Two brothers may no longer be able to talk at length about their favorite sports team. Day-to-day communication becomes increasingly difficult. All of this adds to the challenges of caregiving.

The Best Friends approach has many powerful elements that will enhance communication with people with even advanced stages of dementia. Again, we look to the elements of friendship for inspiration. Good friends communicate in many ways, including verbally and nonverbally. Good friends also make an effort to communicate. Good friends come to understand each other well.

Individuals with Alzheimer's disease or other dementia retain the need to communicate long after their vocabulary and language skills diminish. They want to understand and be understood. However, you as the care partner must also have a desire to communicate with and be present for the person.

BEST FRIENDS PHILOSOPHY OF COMMUNICATION

In good dementia care, it takes a Best Friend to reach out and make a meaningful connection. Here is how it is done.

Remember the Basics of Good Communication

The principles of good communication still apply in dementia care. Communication is enhanced by good eye contact; specific, descriptive language; appropriate volume and tone; and appropriate gestures and body language. However strange it may feel to you, an important first step in approaching a person is to introduce yourself and explain your relationship to him or her, even if you are a family member. When you help out by saying, "Hi Lorraine, it's me, your sister, Mary," you are setting the stage for a positive interaction. Even if she says that she knows who you are and expresses irritation that you have introduced yourself to her, it's possible she didn't really know. Use common sense in these situations but err on the side of better communication.

Nonverbal Communication Paints a Picture

People with dementia are particularly attuned to the care partner's tone of voice, facial expression, volume, and hand gestures. Body language counts! It is as if you are speaking to someone who doesn't speak the same language as you—he or she is looking for cues and clues from the encounter and not relying completely on your spoken words. Examples of positive body language include smiles, offering a handshake, hugs, and standing tall with enthusiasm! Just as important is looking at the person's body language to judge his or her mood. Is she looking worried or anxious, pacing, rubbing her hands, or is she sitting calmly, smiling, and watching the world go by?

The Importance of Positive Body Language

If we need help or are lost and need directions, most of us intuitively look for someone friendly and approachable. A stranger's smile or scowl when you first approach him will determine whether you ask for assistance. The language skills of the person with dementia are diminishing, but he or she can still "read" your face and body language. The person may not understand your words and may not always recognize you, but he or she still recognizes the positive intent of a smile, a handshake, or even an inviting and open posture.

Create an Environment That Facilitates Good Communication

Remember to always consider the environment from the point of view of the person with dementia and how it might inhibit communication. Individuals with memory loss receive messages from everything in their surroundings. Therefore, to aid communication, the environment should be well lit, uncluttered, and pleasant. Be sure it is free of distractions and ambient noise. Try to facilitate interactions in whichever room in the house is most suited to conversation.

Treat the Person as an Adult

Use simple language but keep it adult in nature. "Baby talk" is almost always a bad idea. Likewise, you do not need to speak so slowly that it becomes ridiculous. Also, be aware of and try to avoid the tendency to use the "royal we." To say to the person, "Let's take our medicine" when he or she is the only one taking a pill can be confusing. If you say, "Let's put on our pants," the person might genuinely wonder who will be wearing the pants!

Treating the person as an adult is an important part of maintaining good communication. Adults want to talk about meaningful subjects, engage in activities that are meaningful, and have choices about their lives. For example, one care partner we know wakes his mother up with a nice cup of coffee, discusses the schedule for the day, offers her a simple choice about her clothes for the day, and tries to engage her in a conversation about something in the day's news ("Mom, today is Mark Twain's birthday"). He says he strives for a sense of normalcy that it is calming for both of them.

Maintain Integrity

It is best to start from a position of truth whenever possible when being asked questions by the person or in discussing various situations. People with dementia are often more resilient and flexible than you would imagine. However, if truth telling creates great stress or prevents important tasks from happening, we believe it is ethically permissible to withhold information or to deal with situations with finesse. For example, if the person has lost a set of dentures and refuses to replace them due to the cost (even if he or she has plenty of savings; perhaps the person has a delusion of being broke), you may stretch the truth by saying that "insurance will pay for them." You are doing this for the person's health and best interests, not your own convenience.

Use the Person's Life Story Often

People with dementia can recognize things from their Life Story even when they cannot retrieve the memories on their own. Using the Life Story can enhance communication in all kinds of ways, including providing cues during personal care, enhancing conversations, and helping you prevent challenging behaviors. For example, if your father is refusing to take a shower, you might find that talking about his favorite baseball team and love of old cars might create a better mood and foster cooperation. If your loved one is in a residential care community or day center, it is vitally important that staff know his or her Life Story well if they are to give the best possible care. See Chapter 5 for more on the Life Story.

Respond to Emotional Needs

If the person can articulate concerns or feelings about his or her illness, you should empathize and validate them. ("It must be difficult when you forget things. That happens to me sometimes, too.") It is also important to try to understand the emotion behind unintelligible words. If the person seems upset, you can say, "I'm sorry about that." When he or she seems happy, you can say, "That must have been great!" Touch and hugs can make an emotional connection and provide reassurance.

Remember That Behaviors Communicate a Message

Early in the disease, the person probably can communicate feelings and problems in words; later, his or her behavior articulates what words cannot. If he is yelling or striking out, this can signify that he is in pain or has an infection and needs medical attention. Wandering can suggest boredom. Tears can suggest loneliness and the need for more activity and interaction with other people. When you stop, look, and listen, the person's behaviors communicate many things.

The Best Friends Philosophy of Communication

- Remember the basics of good communication
- Nonverbal communication paints a picture
- Create an environment that facilitates good communication
- Treat the person as an adult
- Maintain integrity
- Use the person's Life Story often
- Respond to emotional need
- Remember that behaviors communicate a message
- Do not take the person too literally
- Employ good timing
- Use repetition to facilitate better communication
- Do not argue or confront
- Screen out troubling messages or news
- Use positive body language
- Use humor in conversation
- Do most of the work

Do Not Take the Person Too Literally

Have patience, and recognize that the disease process affects the person's ability to remember and use words. For example, the person may think he or she is being clear but may be using the wrong word. He or she may say, "Hand me that glass" while really meaning, "Hand me that toothbrush." The person may know who you are but not be able to get the name out correctly. With dementia's attack on the brain's language centers, words, sentence structure, and language are failing.

Employ Good Timing

Good timing is an art. It is always helpful to observe the person's patterns and habits. Is he or she a morning person or a night owl? Knowing this can help you strategize about the best time of day to approach him or her for a bath or other tasks. Good timing also involves patience in speaking and listening. If the person is trying to say something, give him or her time to speak, but do not let the struggle for words go on so long that frustration sets in. If you try to start up a conversation and strike out, don't completely give up. Try again later in the day; you may then find success.

Use Repetition to Facilitate Better Communication

Asking a question twice, with additional descriptive cues for greater emphasis, can help the person better understand what you are saying: "Uncle Matt, hand me that rake [pointing]. Please, Uncle Matt, hand me that green rake over there with the wooden handle [pointing]." In this case, the repetition involves more descriptive language and specific nouns instead of nondescript pronouns ("the rake" versus "it").

Do Not Argue or Confront

It is virtually impossible to win an argument with an individual with dementia. For example, if your mother says President Clinton is doing a good job, ask her to tell you more about that instead of telling her that he is no longer president. Trying to present an argument or to convince the person of a particular point of view will lead to frustration and failure. Also, confrontation will only cause the person to be more defensive, further harming communication.

This means curbing your own defensive reactions when the person makes unjustified accusations or complaints against you. Letting go of the little things and not arguing is one of the most important lessons for successful care.

Screen Out Troubling Messages or News

Individuals with dementia have difficulty sorting information; therefore, it is important to screen out sad, violent, ominous, or controversial messages when possible. Be careful not to listen to television news excessively or talk about negative headlines from the newspaper or websites. Even distressing stories with a happy ending can cause the person to worry. For example, if a neighbor tells him that her dog ran away but was later found, he may still dwell on the first part of the message.

Use Positive Language

People with Alzheimer's disease are often still proud and may resent being told what to do. Whenever possible, speak to the person using positive language. It is better to say, "Let's go this way," than to say, "Don't go that way." Remember that one element of knack is having empathy for the person, to walk a mile in his or her shoes. When we do that, we realize that we would not want to be talked down to or bossed around if we had dementia.

Use Humor in Communication

Sharing humorous moments is communication at its finest. It involves bonding and an emotional release. Consider telling a funny story to the person. While hearing the story, she laughs, smiles, and has a welcoming posture. Her face is animated. She picks up feelings of happiness and the spirit of fun. Also, laughter is infectious; we tend to laugh at a joke whether we "get it" or not.

Do Most of the Work

Because the disease process has an impact on language, you cannot expect the person to do an equal share of the work in conversations. You must keep working to be an effective communicator. Sometimes this is easy and sometimes it is hard, but even a few words and small efforts may trigger remaining skills. A simple phrase that helps is "Tell me more." You can also restate what the person has said and fill in some gaps in conversation to keep things flowing.

LET'S PRACTICE COMMUNICATING WITH KNACK

Care partners with the knack for communicating have empathy and patience, focus on the present, use humor, and attempt to lighten up on life even when things are tough. You can get the knack by using the above techniques to avoid common communication dead ends.

Following are some sample situations to demonstrate the knack of communication in action.

Avoid Arguments

A man with Alzheimer's disease thinks he has a Rotary club meeting today, when in fact he went the day before.

SPOUSE: "Honey, I think you've already been to Rotary this week. Let's check the calendar together. Oh, here it is; you went yesterday. I've been all mixed up myself this week since Monday was a holiday."

It is tempting to want to say to him, "What's wrong with you? Why don't you try harder? You know that lunch was yesterday. You've already gone. You won't go again till next week." However, it's never a good idea to argue, put someone down, or push him or her to do better. Like the wife in the above story, sometimes it is good to "take the blame" or "fall on the sword." She didn't overreact and instead said that she had problems keeping appointments straight as well. They looked at the calendar together, which gently cued him about the correct dates and allayed his concerns. Once again, you can never win an argument with a person with dementia!

Friendly Give and Take

- Don't be afraid to lighten up and enjoy some friendly "give and take" conversations. When words are light and positive, the tone becomes humorous. The person will often see your positive body language and smile and join in the banter.
- Old familiar stories can be used to gently tease someone about something that happened in the past, such as, "I can't believe that we packed the whole family in that station wagon and drove 2,000 miles without air conditioning," or "Did you really put a goat on top of the administration building one Halloween at college?"
- Give-and-take conversation can be spontaneous and simple, such as, "Look at us today. We're dressed just alike." Wait for a response; often the person will respond that you both do look alike. The conversation can continue with, "You are in pink, and so am I. We are both 'in the pink'" (laughing at this old saying that means "everything is okay" or "life is good").

Make Directions Clear

In this example, you can see how an in-home worker encourages his client Lance to enjoy a bowl of soup.

IN-HOME WORKER: [Making eye contact] "Lance, come on. We don't want the tasty chicken soup to get cold."

LANCE: "Where?"

IN-HOME WORKER: [Gestures with hands and speaks in pleasant tone] "Sit with me here in the dining room. Here, sit in the brown chair. [Pats hand on dining room chair, smiling broadly] Come on, we don't want this delicious chicken soup to get cold."

LANCE: "Soup, that sounds good to me."

IN-HOME WORKER: [As Lance sits down] "I'm glad you're here beside me."

Note that the home worker speaks in short, direct sentences. She calls her client by name, repeats key phrases, and uses gestures and body language effectively. Also, she adds emphasis by mentioning the dining room, the brown chair, and the delicious soup awaiting him.

Cope with a Mother's Accusations

It can be quite hurtful when a person makes a false accusation. In this case, the son handles it with calmness and skill.

MOTHER: [Angrily] "You took my purse! Where's my money?"

SON: [Keeps some distance, speaks in a calm voice, looking directly in his mother's eyes] "Mom, it's me, Jeff, your son. You are such a teaser. [Smiles] Let me help you. I bet if we look together for a few minutes we'll find that purse."

MOTHER: "Jeff, someone took my purse."

SON: "Mom, tell me about that purse."

MOTHER: "It's my purse."

SON: "I think I remember that you had the red purse out today. Was it the red purse?"

MOTHER: "Yes."

SON: "Here it is, Mom. You know, I put it in the drawer for safekeeping. I'm very sorry if I upset you. I won't do it again."

MOTHER: "Well, okay. Don't touch it again."

Jeff handles this challenging situation well by keeping his distance initially and letting his mother vent. He introduces himself and then teases his mother a bit, attempting to provide a small distraction. The son says that he had put the purse away for his mother. He has the knack of taking the blame for his mother, smoothing over a difficult situation and helping her "save face."

Understanding Seemingly Incomprehensible Words

Sometimes language abilities are profoundly damaged and the person's words and self-expression don't make much sense. Here is an example of a sister working hard to make the communication connection with her brother who has dementia.

BROTHER: [Looking agitated] "Um, that's out. Cold."

SISTER: [Studies her brother's face, sees concern] "Greg, is something wrong?"

BROTHER: "It's cold. Noise. Cold."

SISTER: "It is cold outside. Let's look out the door. Will you help me take a look? [Takes Greg by the hand and gently leads him to the sliding glass door] Brrr, it is cold out there! Show me what you see."

BROTHER: "Linda, there was noise."

SISTER: "Oh, are you looking at that cat out there? How did Mouser get out? Shall we let him in? He's looking for a warm lap to sit in. I think he likes you best, Greg. Let's call him in and go sit by the fire."

Linda demonstrated effective communication by being patient, treating her brother's concerns as real, and piecing together the clues to discover that the cat had indeed gotten out in cold weather. By studying Greg's body language (his face and pacing), she determined that there was a problem and appropriately responded by asking, "Is something wrong?" Perhaps in this case she may also recall that Greg uses the word "noise" when he refers to the cat's "meow." Greg's beloved Mouser is back in the house safe and sound.

Even if there had been no cat at all, Linda's technique would help Greg feel validated and provide calming reassurance.

Encouraging a Bathroom Stop

Here is a good example of turning a "no" into a "yes." Bathroom behavior is always a bit delicate to discuss, but this son is both specific and sensitive. He employs good timing by repeating the request until he is successful.

SON: [Leaving a restaurant, softly asks] "Dad, do you have to go to the bathroom to pee?"

FATHER: "No."

SON: [Whispers to him] "Let's stop at the bathroom before we go home."

FATHER: "I'm okay."

SON: "Okay, let's leave. [Pats his father on the shoulder, smiling, making a hand gesture toward the front door; as they pass by the men's bathroom door, he says] Dad, let's both go in here for a minute. It's a long way home. I need to go to the bathroom." [Successfully leads him into the men's room]

Often people with dementia will automatically say no to something when they do not quite understand what is being asked of them, or in this case, may not know where the bathroom is. The son showed knack by not embarrassing his father or treating him like a child (he whispered his initial request). Rather than argue, he went ahead and gently coaxed his father again, saying "Let's both go." He turned a "no" into a "yes" by using finesse.

Dealing with Loss

With dementia, the person may forget that a favorite relative or friend has died. Here is one way to manage that situation.

MOTHER: [Maria, looking for her husband, who died two years ago] "Manuel. Where's Manuel? Manuel."

DAUGHTER: "Mom, Dad isn't here. Come with me. Let's have a cup of tea and talk about Dad. I remember the time he restored that Ford Mustang in the garage. You got to pick out the cherry red color!"

Maria and her husband were very close, and she still calls for him occasionally. The daughter knows that it is very upsetting when someone reminds her mother of Manuel's death. Mother forgets being told, but the sadness and distress linger. The daughter does not deny her mother's feelings and instead invites her to spend time talking about her husband.

Earlier in the disease process, Maria probably could have understood, if reminded, that Manuel had died. Later in the illness, care partners must use their own best judgment about whether telling the truth will be helpful and healing or be confusing and overly upsetting.

CONCLUSION

One son we knew decided that one of the best times to practice communicating as a Best Friend was over mealtimes with his mother. He had moved back into the family home to help his frail elderly father and his mother with dementia. Here are some of the "new family traditions" he instituted with great success. With his mother he:

- Encouraged her to help set the table or pour the iced tea. This provided an opportunity for her to feel valued and for the son to give compliments.
- Used positive body language, welcoming her to the table with a friendly smile and hug.
- Began with a familiar prayer to reinforce past rituals and support his mother spiritually.
- Asked his mother open-ended questions: How is the roast beef today? What is the best part of that recipe?
- He used food as an opportunity for reminiscence, asking her to talk about when she first had mashed potatoes or whether her

mother was a good cook, or by introducing opportunities to tell favorite stories: "I remember, Mom and Dad, that you once told me a bear ate all your food when you went camping in Yellowstone! Was that really true?"

- The son used this time for offering reassuring words, such as "Mom, I'm so glad to be having lunch with you. You have on a beautiful sweater today. That purple color looks great on you!"
- He also utilized his mother's Life Story. Because she was raised on an orchard, the son would ask, "Mom, what do you think of these apples? I bet the ones you grew on your farm in Washington tasted better." "When is the best time to pick apples?" "Did you get many wormy ones?"

Heartfelt communication done the Best Friends way supports interactions that can rise above the losses of dementia.

Best Friends Pointers

- Most people have a deeply felt need to communicate. Employ techniques and strategies to help bridge the gap caused by the person's declining communication abilities.
- Encourage conversation by talking about familiar experiences, traditions, and accomplishments from the Life Story.
- Remember the importance of body language. Reassuring gestures, a smile, and a hug can communicate a powerful message to the person that all is well.
- When you can't understand the words, seek to understand the underlying feelings.

8

BEING TOGETHER

Managing and Valuing Activities

Most people engage in activities they enjoy—maybe you play sports, garden, go to a movie, go on a date, read a new mystery novel, go to the gym, surf the Web, play with the dog, or spend time with your family. For many, work is also important; successes on the job and socializing with coworkers make us feel valued. Leisure activities and work provide a sense of identity, community, and self-esteem.

Sadly, the person with Alzheimer's disease and other dementia begins to lose the ability to initiate and be a part of many activities he or she has once enjoyed. This can be a bitter pill for an active individual who now begins to become isolated. And for the care partner, filling the day sometimes can be an ongoing struggle, especially knowing that behaviors that are challenging often rise to the surface if the person is bored. At the same time, family members and friends need to maintain their own interests and activities, which can be difficult if the whole day is consumed with trying to plan activities for the person with dementia. But when the care partner is enjoying the time as a Best Friend, the person senses this shared fun, excitement, or satisfaction. The Best Friends approach to activities should let you attain a balance between the person's needs and yours.

BEST FRIENDS APPROACH TO ACTIVITIES

Learning a new way of approaching activities is a key element in becoming a successful Best Friend. Engaging persons with dementia in everyday life creates opportunities for socialization and in many ways is the "treatment" for dementia. Getting the knack for activities involves grasping the "art of being together." This includes formal and planned activities as well as spontaneous moments. It includes exercise, games, reading, music, and watching old movies. It also includes simple thirty-second interactions such as giving a hug, a short hand massage, a joke, or even a smile. It includes recasting personal care so that a bath can become an opportunity to enjoy the scent of the shampoo, and getting dressed can become a spontaneous fashion show. It includes using the Life Story for reminiscence and touching the spirit through a person's faith beliefs or relationship with nature and the arts. All of us enjoy all of these kinds of "activities" in our daily lives and so should the person with dementia. Ideally, every day includes these elements whether the person is at home, at a day center, or in residential care settings.

The Best Friends approach to activities begins with knowing these basics:

The Art of Activities Is Not in What Is Done, It Is in the Doing

The process of the activity is always more important than the result or end product. If an activity such as folding bath towels is accompanied by smiles, conversation, friendly gossip, discussion about fabrics and colors, and praise for a job well done, it should not matter if the towels are not folded with perfect edges. As the old saying suggests, "It's the journey, not the destination, that counts."

Activities Should Be Individualized and Tap into Past Interests and Skills

Consider the person's Life Story when thinking about activities. A person who enjoyed playing cards, for example, might not be able to play poker or bridge anymore but might enjoy playing a game with assistance, switching to a simpler game, shuffling the deck, checking the deck to find missing cards, or simply being present and watching others play. A person who was always highly organized may enjoy sorting activities such as putting the deck of cards in order by suit or by number.

Activities Should Be Adult in Nature

Activities that are unnecessarily juvenile can provoke frustration, even anger. The person can sense when an activity is demeaning or obviously busy work. Some people with dementia respond positively to dolls or children's toys, but you should not use this fact as an excuse to keep all activities at this level. When doing art-related activities, use colorful pens and markers or brushes, not childlike crayons.

Activities Should Recall a Person's Work-Related Past

Many people with dementia enjoy activities that touch on their work experiences, in part because work played an enormous role in their lives. An artist may want to continue painting. A homemaker may enjoy organizational tasks or a discussion about canning fruits and vegetables. A teacher may enjoy reading about an interesting topic on the Internet.

Activity Pointers

- The art of activities is not in what is done, it is in the doing.
- Activities should be individualized and tap into past interests and skills.
- Activities should be adult in nature.
- Activities should recall a person's work-related past.
- Activities should stimulate all five senses.
- Doing nothing is actually doing something.
- Activities should tap into a person's remaining physical skills.
- Activities should be initiated by others.
- Activities should be voluntary.
- Intergenerational activities are especially desirable.
- Activities you think will never work sometimes do.
- Personal care is an activity.
- Activities can be short.
- Activities are everywhere.
- Activities should fulfill religious and spiritual needs.

Activities Should Stimulate All Five Senses

Although some of the senses are diminished by age, many remain strong. We have found that the most successful activities stimulate more than one sense. For example, gardening involves touching wet soil, smelling different flowers, hearing the crunch of leaves underfoot, tasting fruit off a tree or a tomato off a vine, and seeing vivid colors in a variety of plants.

Baking might involve smelling the spice or vanilla, tasting the batter, kneading the bread, hearing the timer go off, and seeing the beautiful result.

Doing Nothing Is Actually Doing Something

Even good friends enjoy quiet times together, perhaps just sitting in the living room listening to music or watching the world through a picture window. Sometimes the person is content just to be present, observing others at work. Depending on his or her level of dementia, the person may simply enjoy time alone.

Activities Should Tap Into Remaining Physical Skills

Many individuals with dementia remain in remarkably good physical condition. Care partners should take advantage of this by including activities such as walking, doing active chores, or engaging in other physical tasks. Many individuals with dementia still have good hand-eye coordination. This skill can be used to advantage in a variety of enjoyable games including catch, putting a golf ball, or even shooting baskets with the grandchildren.

Recent research has suggested that exercise is good for the brain and may even help delay the onset of Alzheimer's disease. Build exercise into the person's routine since it promotes muscle strength and balance, contributes to fewer falls, fights depression, and is an old skill that many still enjoy. Exercise can easily be enjoyed and done together by the care partner and the person.

Activities Should Be Initiated by Others

Individuals with dementia slowly lose the ability to initiate activities. The well-planned activity will fail if the person cannot get started. With encouragement and assistance, a retired secretary might still enjoy spelling out words with Scrabble letters or filing papers. She might even volunteer to help fold and mail a newsletter at an Alzheimer's Association office. A retired painter may still enjoy painting but may need to be handed the brush and be shown how to stroke the canvas.

Activities Should Be Voluntary

No one should be forced to do something against his or her will, particularly in the realm of activities. Most people with dementia will not do something they do not enjoy or find satisfying. Some care partners find that if they begin an activity in front of the person, he or she may become interested and then take over the task and continue working happily for a period of time.

However, don't immediately give up if the person says no to an activity. One element of caregiving knack is turning a "no" into a "yes." Review Chapter 7 on communication to best communicate with the person and to overcome resistance.

Intergenerational Activities Are Especially Desirable

Intergenerational activities are generally extremely successful. Both generations benefit from the exchange: Many (but not all) individuals with dementia enjoy being able to watch young people playing or doing an activity or being more involved helping young people complete a task or project. Young people often enjoy the attention, affection, and words of encouragement offered by an elder relative with dementia. Many schools now have community service requirements; a whole new group of students have been introduced to dementia care and activities in day centers and residential care as a result of these progressive volunteer programs.

Look for Surprises

Persons can often use overlearned skills (things we've done so many times we don't think about how we do them) such as folding clothes, adding up numbers, setting the table, or greeting friends with a handshake. Sometimes persons will develop new interests, perhaps a newfound enjoyment of country music or opera. He or she may try a craft project or get up and dance—activities that might have been frowned upon before. Look for surprises in the following areas when it comes to planning an activity:

- Music
- Reminiscing
- Creative arts
- Intergenerational experiences
- Social graces

- Physical activity and exercise
- Old skills
- Old sayings and truisms
- Eye-hand coordination
- Rituals—sacred and secular

Activities You Think Will Never Work Sometimes Do

Many families respond to activity ideas by saying their mother or father "would never do that." Similarly, staff working in long-term care settings can be reluctant to try things that may not succeed. When we began work in adult day centers, we were also rather conservative in our activity programming. We soon learned, however, that people with dementia are full of surprises. A previously shy man who was never a joiner may now be the life of the party. Someone who was never religious may now enjoy an interfaith service. Someone who has never painted may become happily engaged in a watercolor art activity. It is good to question expectations now and then and try new things.

Personal Care Is an Activity

Families should recognize that some of the most difficult personal care chores can become easier when knack is applied. Care partners can take a few extra moments while helping a person bathe or dress to talk about old times, smell a new scented soap, or tell a joke. This puts the person at ease, thus relaxing him or her and making it easier for the care partner to complete the task.

Activities Can Be Short

Often the person's attention span makes it difficult for him or her to be involved in an extended activity. Even very brief activities, repeated often, can fill a day. One care partner would have her father read a number of short poems throughout the day. Another would ask her mother to sweep the kitchen floor. Even if these activities only last a minute or two, a care partner can develop a repertoire of short activities that can effectively be put to use during the day.

Activities Are Everywhere

With knack, almost everything can become an extended, interesting activity. A simple handshake, for example, can lead to a discussion about fingernail polish, gloves, work done by hand, "life lines," rings on fingers, weddings, and more. A teapot can be enjoyed for its beauty; discussions can follow about making tea, reading tea leaves, the different flavors of tea, and the Boston Tea Party.

Touring the Inside

As familiar as everything in your home may seem, you might be surprised how many sources of conversation and discovery it contains for the person with dementia. If the person has lots of energy to expend before going to bed, gets up during the night, or needs a distraction to get him or her down the hall to the bathroom, this activity can be helpful.

Invite the person to join you on an evening walkabout. As you tour the house, stop and look at objects around you. Help the person make connections between what you are seeing and past associations from the person's life. Here are just a few ideas:

- Stop to watch tropical fish in the fish tank.
- Look at the décor and discuss how well the furnishings are arranged.
- Study a painting on the wall. Discuss the subject matter, colors, and technique. Admire the gold-leaf frame. Ask if the painting reminds the person of anything.
- Count the flowers on a potted plant. Wipe the dust off the leaves.
- Reminisce about when different objects in a knick-knack collection were acquired.
- Search for the cat.
- Stop in the kitchen and enjoy the aroma of the coffee grounds. Discuss the pleasure of the next day's cup of fresh coffee.
- Review the notes on the refrigerator or bulletin board.

THE PURPOSE OF ACTIVITIES

In the quest to fill the day for individuals with dementia, it is easy to forget to put the meaning into activities and remember that people like to do things that meet a variety of purposes and needs. Keep the following needs in mind when aiming to fill the person's day.

Be Productive or Make a Contribution

Most of us have a need to feel that we have made a difference to someone's life or to the life of a community. Maybe we are good at our jobs. Maybe we volunteer at a charity. Maybe we are good parents or good friends to others. People with dementia also retain a desire to help, to feel a part of the world. Encourage your family member to do a daily chore or continue to volunteer at the local animal shelter or in his or her faith community as long as possible. Activities can help individuals with memory loss meet this need to feel competent and useful.

Experience Successes

Activities can lead to big and small successes. Many children take pride in assembling a model. A couple who plants a garden together can be proud of their accomplishment and enjoy the compliments from neighbors. People with dementia have faced many losses. Activities as simple as helping bake a cake, brush the dog, or dry the dishes help them enjoy new successes.

Play

Many people spend their lives working hard, so activities can be a place to lighten up and have fun. Individuals with dementia often retain the ability to enjoy playing. They can still tease, joke, and engage in activities such as flying a kite, tossing a ball, or playing a simple video game.

Be with Others

People participate in activities to be with friends, to meet new people, to be part of a club, or simply to feel a part of society. Attending a farmers' market, for instance, can delight with its colorful fruits and vegetables, the smell of food, and the sounds of enjoyable music. Even though individuals with dementia usually feel more comfortable in smaller group settings, they still have the need to belong.

Build Skills

We take part in society and do things to practice what we do well, sharpen old skills, or develop new ones. People with Alzheimer's disease and other dementia may not necessarily be developing new skills, but activities like completing a simple craft project, sanding a piece of wood, or organizing the contents of a drawer can help them renew old skills and practice and preserve remaining skills.

Have a Sense of Control

All of us hope to have some control over our lives. Appropriate activities can help people feel empowered and in charge of their world. People with dementia benefit from feeling a sense of control. For example, some families involve the person in simple financial transactions such as signing checks after the checks have been filled out. When helping a person get dressed, you can ask him what color sweater he wants to wear or offer a simple choice—for example, wearing the brown shoes or black shoes today.

Feel Safe and Secure

All of us have a need for safety and security. If you live in a dangerous neighborhood, fear losing your job, or worry about money, these concerns can create stress and strain. Individuals with dementia have a great need to feel secure and safe from moment to moment. Often, it is simple things, such as enjoying a cup of hot cocoa, helping put the grandchildren to bed, reading a religious text or singing a hymn, or simply sharing a warm hug that recall warm feelings associated with past good times and help reassure the person that all is well.

Fill Religious or Spiritual Needs

Although not everyone professes a religious faith, we believe that everyone has a spiritual life. Individuals with dementia still may have religious or spiritual needs that can be fulfilled in ways that are meaningful to them. Attending religious services or praying may meet the needs of one person, while writing poetry, creating art, walking in a forest, or showing compassion for others may especially touch the spirit of another. Read more about spirituality and dementia in Chapter 9.

Experience Growth and Learning

Many people take part in activities to learn more about a particular subject or for human growth. People with dementia may or may not be able to learn new information, but they still can enjoy the experience of being presented interesting new material. Satisfaction and pleasure come from participating in a learning situation.

SUCCESSFUL ACTIVITIES IN DEMENTIA CARE

When thinking about activities for people with Alzheimer's disease and other dementia, think about what you like to do and why you like to do it—it may fulfill the same need for the person. Below are some activities that we have found successful. Use them as a springboard for your own creativity, and, of course, individualize the activity whenever possible. The following activities can be done almost anywhere, at any time, with few materials or little money. Activities really are everywhere.

Performing Personal Care

Try turning the sometimes daunting tasks of personal care into activities:

- Dressing can become a fashion show.
- Brushing teeth can become a taste test for new toothpaste.
- Combing hair can become an opportunity for a quiet sing-along.
- Toileting can be a time to provide extra reassurance.
- Giving a manicure can be a time to compliment the person.
- Eating a meal can be a time to ask for an opinion.

Bathing as an Activity

For people without dementia, bathing is very often a pleasant, relaxing activity. For people with dementia and their care partners, however, bathing is often more of a "wrestling match" than a soothing activity. Here are some recommendations on how to minimize this daily or continuing struggle and make bathing a more successful activity:

- Think about who the bath is intended to benefit: Does the person really need one or is taking a daily bath just habit or custom?
- Use finesse for a reason to bathe: Are visitors coming? Do you have a special event to go to?
- Who is the person most comfortable to be with during the bath? Spouse, son or daughter, or a hired in-home helper?
- What term is the person most familiar with? Bath? Shower? Washing up?
- When does the person like to be bathed? Morning or evening?
- Is the bathing room inviting, warm, and comfortable?

- Consider how private the person is: Can you find ways to keep the person partially covered?
- Know whether the person prefers a tub bath, shower, or sponge bath? You do not have to use a tub or shower to be completely clean.
- Does the person have a fear of water?
- Let the person help with the bath in some way: Can the person wash his or her own face or hold the washcloth?
- Consider alternatives to traditional bathing: Can the person bathe in places other than the bathroom? Does the person respond better to rinseless soap or a partial bath over several days? Can you jump in the shower with the person (you can be undressed or in a swimsuit)?
- Explore whether using music, reminiscing, or a favorite snack provides a distraction during the bath.
- Offer a special treat for after the bath: Does the person especially like tea and cookies, a drive or outing?

Note: We recommend the book by Barrick et al., *Bathing Without a Battle,* for more advice on this topic. See Organizations, Websites, and Recommended Readings, page 283.

Doing Chores

Help individuals with Alzheimer's disease feel productive with tasks that mimic the satisfaction they received during their working lives:

- Gardening can become a fun family activity.
- Polishing the dining room table can make someone feel useful.
- Folding clothes can keep hand-eye coordination intact.
- Drying dishes can evoke early family memories.

- Raking leaves can be good exercise.
- Sorting through old neckties can evoke the skill of counting.

Being with Pets

Involve the person with friendly family or neighborhood animals and pets if the person enjoys such contacts.

- Listening to the singing of a bird can provide an impromptu concert.
- Brushing a dog can be an opportunity to give and receive unconditional love.
- Holding a cat in the lap lets the person enjoy its soothing purr.
- Feeding ducks can be a highlight of a relaxing, sunny afternoon in the park.
- Schooling tropical fish provides a kaleidoscope of colors.
- Giving the person some responsibility for pet care can make him or her feel needed and build self-esteem.

Using the Magic of Music

Know that music is the language of Alzheimer's disease. Song lyrics, for example, remain intact much longer than a person's ability to converse.

- Listening to the music channels on cable, satellite television, or Internet radio can become a daily tradition after lunch and allow the care partner to get some chores accomplished. Attending a church choral concert can be a chance to dress up in fancy clothes.

- Listening to the person's favorite music in the car can add comfort and fun to a trip.
- Tapping fingers and toes to a pronounced rhythm can provide the person with exercise.
- Dancing cheek-to-cheek can be romantic.
- Holding a whistling contest can make everyone laugh.
- Moving to rhythmic music can reduce anxiety and be an excuse for some exercise.

Reminiscing

Encourage reminiscing; it fulfills a basic human need to think about the past.

- Enjoying the aroma of a bottle of perfume can evoke memories of getting dressed for a dinner party.
- Examining advertisements of kitchen appliances in an old magazine or from images printed from the Internet can be a fun activity and can lead to talk about an old remodeling project or one's first kitchen.
- Looking at framed pictures displayed on the bookshelf can lead to comparisons between then and now.
- Handling ribbons and wrapping paper and wrapping gifts can prompt a discussion about favorite presents and past birthday parties.
- Listening to a Beatles song can bring back memories of college days in the 1960s and 1970s.
- Comparing old and new baby clothes can produce smiles and tears of joy.

Remembering Old Sayings, Clichés, or Rhymes

Reciting old sayings, clichés, or rhymes can be a source of pleasure.

- Reviewing fill-in-the-blank flash cards of old sayings can be a pleasurable game for the person: "Necessity is the mother of ____________________" or "It's raining cats and _________."
- Matching rhymes, such as *glad* and *sad* or *post* and *toast*, can engage a person who is worried or anxious.
- Teasing with old sayings can encourage a person to get something done: "A bird in the hand is worth two in the bush."
- Sharing classic poems can be an opportunity to read together for enjoyment or even for the person to recall and recite portions memorized in school.
- Using similes related to animals, such as *loose as a goose* or *naked as a jaybird*, can cause even the most serious person to laugh.
- Reading nursery rhymes aloud can allow the person to "teach" something new to children.

Playing Word Games

Recognize that vocabulary learned long ago can be retrieved through clever word games. Here are some activities that work well in group settings or as part of a small family gathering:

- Naming opposites—up and down, top and bottom, right and left—can be played to fill time at a doctor's office, during a trip, or during other potentially stressful times.
- Listing every word with a certain color, such as Red Sea, red sky, red flag, red-handed, and redhead, can allow persons with dementia to participate in group activities.

- Composing a get-well card together can fulfill the need to help others.
- Using Scrabble letters to spell out key words from the person's past can be a way to honor the person's life story and touch on past achievements.
- Naming state capitals can be a pleasurable memory game.
- Guessing the answers to a trivia game can be an activity the whole family enjoys.

Fun with Old Sayings

Old sayings remain a popular activity for persons with dementia. Because these old sayings are so familiar, they seem to remain in the memory longer than other words or phrases. Here are some fun old sayings about animals. Read the first half aloud and ask the person with dementia to complete the saying. Then enjoy a brief discussion about the saying. For example, you can start out saying, "You can't teach an old dog . . ." and then let the person respond, "new tricks." Then enjoy a short discussion. Is that saying true?

Use the Internet to learn more about the origins of these old sayings:

- Birds of a feather flock together.
- A bird in the hand is worth two in the bush.
- Curiosity killed the cat.
- Dog days of summer.
- You can lead a horse to water but you can't make it drink.
- The early bird gets the worm.
- Don't look a gift horse in the mouth.
- Pig in a poke.
- Bats in the belfry.

- Snake eyes.
- Whale of a good time.
- More fun than a barrel of monkeys.
- Raining cats and dogs.
- Kill two birds with one stone.
- Like a chicken with its head cut off.
- The best laid plans of mice and men.
- The straw that broke the camel's back.
- Don't count your chickens before they hatch.
- Get your ducks in a row.
- What's good for the goose is good for the gander.
- Loose as a goose.
- A leopard can't change its spots.
- Taking the bull by the horn.
- The cat's meow.

From *The Best Friends Book of Alzheimer's Activities, Volume 1*, © 2004, Health Professions Press. Used with permission.

Doing Activities with Children

Remember that children can be especially loving and accepting of people with dementia. Intergenerational activities can bring much joy to persons by letting them feel they are helping or teaching young people.

- Making a Halloween mask together can involve both individuals in a fulfilling art project.
- Reading stories aloud to one another can be an opportunity for praise.

- Walking together can provide exercise and a chance to pick wildflowers.
- Enjoying the festivities surrounding a common birthday—blowing out candles, exchanging presents, singing "Happy Birthday," and eating birthday cake—can evoke smiles and laughter.
- Being with children can make it acceptable for adults to play childlike games and work simple puzzles.
- Receiving the hugs and kisses children give so freely makes the person feel loved.

Community Activity Ideas

Go for a drive.

Sit on a park bench.

Attend a religious service.

Visit your favorite ice-cream parlor.

Practice golf at the driving range.

Enjoy a farmer's market.

Walk in the mall.

Visit a friend.

Go to the zoo.

Attend an exhibit at an art museum.

Swim in the neighborhood pool.

Run errands together.

Attend a granddaughter's soccer game.

Attend a class together.

Get to know other couples or families coping with dementia.

Enjoying Quiet Time

Design time for quiet reflection or watching the world go by. This kind of quiet time can calm the person and help the care partner recharge his or her batteries.

- Visiting the library to flip through all the latest magazines in a quiet, studious atmosphere can often be calming to the person.
- Starting a new tradition of afternoon "high tea" and cookies can build a daily ritual.
- Planning a daily walk focuses the person on a single task and can be equally enjoyed by the care partner.
- Taking a drive down a country road can be a chance to be outdoors.
- Watching hummingbirds sip nectar from flowers can help the person connect with nature.
- Sitting quietly in a church or synagogue can be comforting.

Performing Spiritual Activities

Celebrate the religious or spiritual background of the person you care about.

- Reading aloud from the Bible or other religious texts can be reassuring.
- Celebrating religious holidays can help a person feel connected.
- Involving the person in helping a local charity can help him or her feel compassion for others.
- Continuing to attend religious services can help a person feel valued.
- Seeing a beautiful sunrise can lift a person's spirit and make him or her feel more attuned to the universe.

- Looking at large picture books of famous paintings or visiting a museum can touch a person's spiritual side.

Recognizing Old Skills

Take special note of old skills and encourage the person to continue to use them as much as possible.

- Reading aloud from the newspaper can support adult learning and feelings of success.
- Reciting the Gettysburg Address or some other memorized speech or poem can create a successful moment.
- Playing marbles (with a child) gives permission to play.
- Writing e-mails or responding to them can help a person feel connected with family and friends.
- Cooking fried green tomatoes or another special dish can celebrate a person's heritage.
- Spinning a top is an old skill that can be easily taught to others.
- Completing a simple crossword puzzle can be a good after-breakfast project.

Using Creative Arts and Crafts

Understand that many arts and crafts provide an opportunity for the person to utilize remaining strengths and abilities.

- Drawing or painting a memory from childhood, such as a house or school, can help a person feel connected to his or her past.
- Recognizing familiar paintings in an oversized art book helps a person feel competent.
- Using clay to sculpt an animal stimulates the senses.

- Assembling a mobile from objects gathered on an impromptu scavenger hunt (pine cones, leaves, and feathers) evokes old artistic skills.
- Covering oranges with dried cloves to give as gifts is a rich sensory experience.
- Designing decorations for a holiday party involves group socialization.

Evaluating Activities in Professional Settings

If you have a choice of day centers or residential communities, choose the one that is activity rich. A simple way to evaluate the activities is to ask yourself whether you would enjoy the activities if you were in the program. Does the program have a signature activity or show creativity with its activity programming? The best activities should stimulate the senses, involve physical exercise, be outdoors when the weather is nice, or involve music and the arts.

Activities should also be individualized, taking into account the Life Stories of individuals in the facility or day center. You should not see bingo played every day or an overreliance on crafts. Most persons have focused on work as much or more than play in their lives. Activities need to be more than fun and games to hold the interest of many people with dementia.

If you are interviewing home-care companies, ask if they train their in-home workers on the importance of activities. While you may be looking for help with chores and personal care, you also want someone who will engage the person in conversation and meaningful activities that will build a caring relationship.

CONCLUSION

The activities in this chapter are just starting points. Certainly, there are many more activities that can be done with almost no materials or money and on the spur of the moment. Many traditional resources or activities fail because they focus on recipes for activities instead of the *process* of activities. Remember that the secret of the Best Friends philosophy is that it is not necessarily *what* you do—it is the *doing*.

Here is a great example shared by a care partner at a support group:

> *This man had a tradition of bringing his mother a fresh bouquet of flowers every Saturday after he went to his local farmers' market. She always lit up when he brought the arrangement to her assisted living apartment. One day he was late going to the market and all the prearranged bouquets were sold, so he purchased three bunches of different flowers. When he got to his mother's apartment, he apologized and offered to help her arrange them. An hour slipped by as they talked, figured out which flowers would go where in the vase, and discussed the scents of the flowers and their colors. He realized that always bringing the prearranged bunch was a mistake. By bringing flowers that needed to be cut, handled, and arranged, he and his mother had a project to do together. Now, she smiled not only because she enjoyed the flowers he'd brought, but also because of the feeling of accomplishment from arranging them. As he left for the day, the son complimented his mother: "Mom, no one does it better than you do. You did a great job with this flower arrangement! They're beautiful and so are you."*

Best Friends Pointers

- The best activities are ones the person enjoys and finds meaningful.
- Activities need not be long, planned ones. They can be spontaneous and last only a few minutes.
- If you think of personal care as an activity, it is often easier to complete the task.
- A good way to evaluate a day center or residential care program is by the activities. Would you enjoy them if you were in the program? Will your family member enjoy them?
- When employing in-home workers, assess if they will do more than chores and personal care. Will they engage the person in meaningful, relationship-building activities?

9

INNER PASSAGE

Spiritual Journeying and Religion

Often family members ask what happens to their loved one's spiritual life or religious convictions when Alzheimer's disease and other dementia strikes. Can he still be religious if he cannot remember passages from the Bible, prayers, and other traditions and rituals he cherished? Can she retain her spiritual connection to nature even if she becomes homebound? We believe that the answer is yes.

Dr. James Holloway had a doctorate in philosophy from Yale University. When he was asked for his definition of spirit, he no longer could give a formal, academic answer, as he once might have done, because of his dementia. Instead he quickly responded, "That's a tough one! Well, I can tell you one thing, it's not what a lot of people think it is. It is not something far off. It is what keeps us going."

We particularly like his last phrase, "It is what keeps us going." Food to stave off hunger or shelter to stay warm at night is essential to life. Yet it is our quest for meaning, place, and purpose in our lives that defines us as human beings. Many individuals embrace formal religious beliefs and practices for their spiritual connection. Others meet their spiritual needs in other ways, such as through the visual arts, music, or nature.

Just as those with dementia may need help getting dressed, they need help fulfilling basic spiritual needs. A person with dementia is usually unable to attend Mass if no one is available to drive him or her there. Someone with dementia who loves the outdoors may be confined on the third floor of an assisted living community, unable to soak in the sun and hear the birds sing. An artist may not be able to initiate the act of picking up paints and a brush.

A pioneer in dementia care, Tom Kitwood, PhD, pointed out that our role as care partners is to be "physicians of the human spirit." Rather than allow the person with dementia to become spiritually bereft, it is important to treat the human spirit, to open opportunities for spiritual needs to be met. We do this by creating a spiritual space or spiritual moment for the person. This chapter shares ideas to help you do this.

Celebrate the Person's Religious Heritage

Many people with dementia have been members of a religious tradition since early childhood. They have attended religious services, been taught in educational sessions, sung in choirs, visited the sick as representatives of their faith community, and even been religious leaders in their communities. This connection to others and to their

God or a supreme being has helped give meaning and purpose to their lives. Dementia does not negate this even if the person does not fully understand or remember the details of his or her religious practices.

The person with early-stage dementia can participate fully, with a little help as needed, in the life of his or her religious community. The person can stay connected with the community by attending worship services, participating in social occasions, delivering meals to shut-ins with a friend, and maintaining participation in the choir.

Just because Claralee Arnold was having difficulty with her recent memory was no reason for her to give up a cherished activity. She had sung in her church choir since graduation from college. She could still read music, and she loved her friends in the choir. Every Sunday morning, Claralee processed down the aisle in her choir robe and took her place in the choir loft.

Not only did this weekly experience fulfill Claralee's need to be connected to her religious tradition, it also gave further meaning to her life as she used her musical ability to help others.

Families have shared with us the ways their family members with dementia have gotten the most fulfillment from their religious faith:

- Singing and listening to familiar hymns and other religious music.
- Reading or having another read to them from the Bible, Torah, Koran, or other sacred writings.
- Praying or participating in prayers given by another.

- Sharing in religious rituals or traditions, such as the Eucharist or a Seder meal.
- Holding religious symbols such as the cross or prayer beads.
- Lighting the menorah.

These religious activities can be enjoyed at the place of worship or wherever the person is living—in his or her own home or in a residential community. As the dementia progresses, you need to be creative and choose only those things that still seem to help the person connect to his or her faith.

Many families despair when a person can no longer actively participate in religious practices. The best answer to this, we think, came from a caregiver support group member who simply said that in her view, "God is compassionate and caring, particularly for those who are most in need."

Uncovering Comforting Traditions

Josephine, a Catholic woman with advanced dementia, often sat with her eyes closed and made vocal sounds that were difficult to understand, said Dorothy Seman, Assistant Manager of Home Care Programs at the Jesse Brown VA Medical Center in Chicago. While Josephine made these sounds, she moved her hands in a repetitive circular motion. Staff were puzzled until someone ventured, "If I didn't know better, I'd say she was praying the rosary." The next time Josephine made the hand movements, a staff member placed a rosary in her hands. Josephine began fingering the beads. With tears in her eyes, she beamed at the staff member and put the crucifix to her lips to kiss it. Connecting her to her faith and this ritual gave her comfort.

Look to the Creative Arts

The creative arts—think of Mozart's music or Picasso's transforming paintings—take us away from the mundane and allow us to reflect on our lives and our place in the universe. Such expressions of human creativity are part of what makes us spiritual beings. Humans have been creating like this for centuries: Ancient peoples painted caves and decorated their food pots. Later, there was poetry and theater.

Painting, drawing, sculpting, and enjoying the arts fulfills a need for creative expression. In fact, Bruce Miller, MD, Director of the University of California at San Francisco Memory and Aging Center, found that individuals with certain types of dementia can return to an earlier age when creativity and imagination are not discouraged by adult society.

Dancing, rhythmic movement, playing a musical instrument, even simply tapping a beat are all activities that can touch the spirit. One care partner we met took up African drumming, which helped her feel part of a creative community while pounding out her frustration!

Letch Dixon is a clogger. When he hears the beat of the music his feet begin to move. Though his conversation ability is very impaired, he can't stay seated. At the day center he is the first one on his feet. He exudes great joy and a sense of accomplishment. Music is a language that he can understand.

Music and dancing have been part of a spiritual life since the early days of civilization. Today, music and dancing continue to touch the spirit of persons like Letch.

One group of people with dementia spent almost an hour studying an oversized print of the Mona Lisa. Most recognized the image but only one or two could name the work. The group leader asked what they thought of the famous smile. One woman said that someone must have told a joke. A man said that she must be in love. Asked if they thought Mona Lisa was beautiful, they all agreed, "Yes, oh yes." The arts can reach out and touch a person with dementia.

Patricia Estill had always loved to paint and draw. As her losses piled up with things she could no longer do, her love of painting remained. Her spirit seemed to soar to counteract her cognitive decline. Even though her art style changed, her interest in painting endured almost to the end of her life.

Painting fulfilled the need of Patricia's spirit to be productive and important, and her folk art helped her celebrate her African-American heritage.

The Museum of Modern Art (MoMA) in New York City has developed a wonderful program that uses the arts to engage persons with dementia. Many other local museums have created similar programs. Read more about it at http://www.moma.org/meetme/.

Marvel at the Wonders of Nature

Many persons feel spiritually fulfilled when they have the opportunity to spend time in the great outdoors. There they can smell the aroma of blossoms, feel the gentle breeze, hear bird calls, touch the soil as they prepare for a garden plot, and see a squirrel scamper up a tree. We often overlook this longing of some persons to be connected with nature as they may have been all of their lives.

Richard Thompson, a volunteer in the Best Friends Day Center, wrote, "On a beautiful autumn day my Best Friend, John Lackey, and I went for an outside walk with the assigned goal of taking photos to include in his memory book. I first took several snapshots of him using a traditional backdrop beside a water fountain. Then I handed the camera to him. His focus was on cloud formations, tree shapes, the interplay of a jet stream and the sun's rays coinciding with the roofline of a church, and shadows playing in the sunlight. He came 'to life' in a way I had not observed before."

John's wife shared with us that John had always loved being with nature and could always spot a special sunset and gather the family for a "sunset alert." They had spent time in state and national parks and hiked as a family on family vacations. This experience was just another expression of John's lifelong love of nature.

Richard continues: "While my focus had been on the ordinary, John soared to breathtaking views that I would have missed, totally, had he not been directing my attention in a different direction. I learned from this day's project that dementia does not rob all of one's capabilities at the same time. His artist perspective was very much alive and appreciated but I also learned just how limited my own observational skills had become. I look up more often now thanks to my Best Friend."

For some persons, being able to marvel at the created world fulfills a great spiritual need and we, as friends, can learn to "look up" more often.

Being with Friends and Family

Most of us gain tremendous feelings of connection and community from being with our friends and families. These loved ones know our stories, values, and beliefs. We celebrate traditions together. We do things together. We talk. Being with friends and family is an important part of a spiritual life.

Persons with dementia can become isolated and denied this key element of a spiritual life. We want to create opportunities for them to enjoy being with friends and family in a space that encourages communication. For example, it can touch the spirit for a person with dementia to do a simple activity one-on-one with a family member (like arranging flowers), say a prayer or spiritual reading together, enjoy some beautiful music, or simply take time for a walk outside.

Dorothy Troxel loved being with friends and family. On special occasions, the table would be set with Dorothy's beautiful china dishes, fresh flowers, and lovely tablecloth. Dorothy would "host a tea" for her friends and family and enjoy this old ritual.

Sometimes friends and family feel uncomfortable visiting a person with dementia, not knowing what to do or what not to do. Encourage friends and family to continue their visits and just to be in the moment and not worry about the outcome. Stress that the person enjoys our presence and plan for a simple activity like the tea party to make the experience more enjoyable for all.

Nourish Your Own Spiritual Life

Caregiving can be a difficult job, and sometimes the most caring and involved family and staff members burn out the fastest. One way to avoid burnout is to take care of your own spiritual needs. Spiritual self-care can involve maintaining your own faith traditions, taking time to keep a journal, playing a musical instrument, or being outdoors. Many individuals with a religious tradition view their work as care partners as one way to show God's love.

Tap Steven and his wife, Frankie, participate in music and singing. Tap also writes poetry about his life and condition out of the strong need to help others who may be going through a similar experience. Although they feel his Alzheimer's-related losses, both believe that they are living life to the fullest and celebrating their spiritual values in their everyday lives.

Another way to nourish your own spiritual needs is to seek personal support from your faith community. Many communities have a "minister of aging concerns" who focuses on older members.

Because of the slow and progressive nature of Alzheimer's disease and other dementia, it may be harder for others in your faith community to recognize your problems and needs. If your faith community is not knowledgeable about dementia and care partner needs, invite a speaker to give a talk or ask if a support group can be started on-site.

Spiritual self-care also involves time spent thinking about issues such as grief and loss, death and dying. You might find it helpful to find a counselor who specializes in this area.

Alternatives to Regular Religious Services

- Attend part of the service (prayers, readings, music, meaningful rituals).
- Attend a smaller, more informal worship service, class, or social gathering.
- Attend special services, especially musical programs or events celebrating a religious holiday.
- Visit the place of worship when no service is being held; just to sit in the "holy space."
- Watch a religious service or program on television or the Internet.

Give Spiritual Care Throughout the Illness

Individuals with early-stage dementia need as much independence as possible and are often able to fulfill many of their own needs.

Phil Zwicke's Alzheimer's disease did not keep him from his passion for the ocean. He loved windsurfing in the Santa Barbara channel. This put him in touch with the sea, with dolphins and whales, with the blue sky and breeze. It brought him comfort and peace.

As the disease progresses, there may be less and less that a person can do. Many faith communities have staff or volunteers who participate in visitation programs, bringing all or part of the services or rituals to your loved one at home or in a residential care community. If your loved one is at a day center or residential program, be sure to give staff members ideas about what is meaningful to him or her.

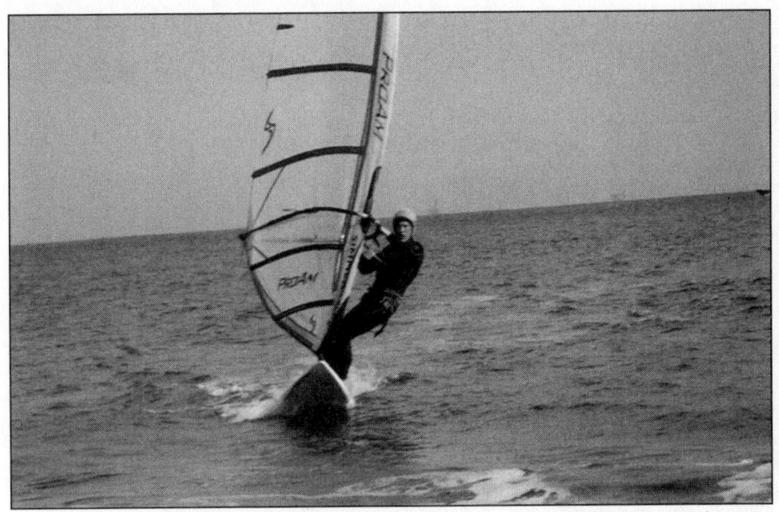

Phil Zwicke still enjoying one of his favorite activities.

Annie Holman gradually became unable to attend the church where she had been very active all of her life. But she enjoyed listening to favorite hymns, seeing a smile, feeling a touch, and hearing her name called. It seemed to connect her to the love she had known in her church community.

Ways to provide spiritual care at the end of life will vary from person to person. You are the most likely to know what will be most helpful to the person. Does your mother smile when you tell her you love her? Does she seem at peace when her minister prays with her? Does she respond when you hold her hand? Does she enjoy hearing favorite religious songs? Does she come to life when the great-grandchildren come for a visit? Does she know that someone who loves her is present? Sensitive, loving care at the end of life is essential for the person and for you.

Many families take advantage of hospice services at the end of the person's life. Most hospices provide spiritual support and counseling during this difficult time.

The Power of Quietness

"It's important to provide quiet times of reflection in addition to outward socialization," says Leslie Congleton, Program Coordinator for Legacy Health Systems' Trinity Place Alzheimer's Day Respite Program in Portland, Oregon. "So often professionals who are involved with providing activities for individuals with dementia focus on the outward, social, upbeat party times and neglect the thirst that each of us has for quiet inward times."

From *The Best Friends Staff: Building a Culture of Care in Alzheimer's Programs*, © 2002, Health Professions Press. Used with permission.

Embrace Simplicity

A person with dementia faces a shrinking world. The international banker now organizes his desk drawer once an hour. The gourmet cook now can only stir and taste the soup. Although most people despair these losses, they often reach a point in the disease when their needs change and they begin to take pleasure from simple, repetitive tasks. These tasks can connect them with something larger than themselves and can hold spiritual meaning.

Edith Hayes had always loved looking for four-leaf clovers. She wrote notes to family and friends for all special occasions and often enclosed a pressed four-leaf clover for good luck. Eventually she could not keep up with her note writing, but she still delighted in searching a clover patch for a prized lucky clover. This simple activity connected her with her spiritual need to find a gift to give others.

Other acts of simplicity celebrate the magic and power of children; many people with dementia enjoy the naiveté and simplicity of children (who also may not be able to name the president of the United States). Sitting on the sofa, listening to classical music may feed the spirit. A simple, familiar prayer or sacred reading can comfort a distressed person with dementia.

CONCLUSION

A common cry of many with dementia is "I want to go home. I want to go home." We believe that this is much more than a literal statement of place and instead is a cry for spiritual connectedness. Home represents a happier time and a place safe from the present and from dementia.

As a care partner, you can create a spiritual space or moment for the person, one that allows the person to "go home" spiritually, if not physically. When loving care is given, it allows people to make their own connection, however limited, to the world of the spirit. When families value the person, a home can become a spiritual space. When care is good and the staff is well trained, a nursing home can become a spiritual space.

When you create this space by offering enhanced activities and a life-affirming environment, something else happens: You create a spiritual space not only for the person with dementia but also for yourself.

One care partner told us this beautiful story at a conference:

Mom and I were taking a walk, and as hard as I tried to be attentive, my mind was on my own problems. I was thinking about work, a problem in my marriage, and some financial decisions. My mother suddenly said, "Look at that!" I looked up toward a group of trees and could see nothing. She said, "Look at that beautiful blue bird." I still couldn't see it. Finally, as I scanned the tree limbs it was there. This incident made me reflect on my mother's world and my own. Now, she always finds the beautiful birds in the trees or smells the scent of flowers in the air and hears music in the distance—all of these things I had shut out. Her Alzheimer's disease has somehow put her back in touch with nature and her spiritual side. I had perfect cognition, but I wasn't seeing any of the world around me. Maybe there are still some things I could learn from her.

Being present is a profound, spiritual gift we can give the person with dementia.

Ironically, the stripping away of cognition actually seems to increase the person's spiritual awareness and might make it easier for us to recognize, understand, and meet the needs of the spirit. The person with dementia may now have an enhanced awareness of and appreciation for familiar religious symbols or icons, a beautiful sunset, music, or art. When you take time to reflect on spirituality, take time to be in the present; the very things that nourish the person with dementia may nourish you as well.

Best Friends Pointers

- Every person has a spirit and is spiritual, whether or not he or she is part of a religious tradition.
- Try to keep the person who has been a member of a faith community connected to those religious practices for as long as possible.
- Look for ways the person finds meaning and purpose in his or her life outside the framework of formal religion, such as in art, nature, music, and friends and family.
- By being a Best Friend to the person with dementia, you will be practicing spiritual care at its best.

10

FINDING HELP

Navigating the Journey

"Caregiving is a life interrupted," states Mynga Futrell, a writer and former care partner. For many families this statement rings true. You can "press the start button" and move this interrupted life forward, however, by taking steps to become a well-informed, proactive care partner. The experience of caring for a person with Alzheimer's disease or other dementia can end up being an opportunity to build a closer relationship with the person, learn new skills, meet new people, and experience a sense of success about the meaningful work you have accomplished.

One key to a successful caregiving experience is finding and using appropriate help. Don't fall into the trap of believing it is all up to you. Today there are many valuable services and programs that can help you travel the journey with your family member or friend with Alzheimer's disease or other dementia. From adult day center programs, to in-home workers, to residential care programs, to end-of-life hospice care, many programs now train their staff members about how to provide excellent care for persons with dementia.

Knowing what each type of service involves and asking the right questions can help you navigate what seems to be a maze of services and help you make good choices for your loved one and for yourself. Using services wisely can also be the difference between success and failure as a care partner. A few hours of help here and there can keep you rested and energized, while offering opportunities for socialization and support to the person.

CARE IN THE HOME

Most care for people with Alzheimer's disease and other dementia takes place in the home. At home, the person can enjoy a familiar chair, wear all of his or her favorite clothes, and play with a beloved pet. Individuals living at home are much more likely to see old friends and participate in community events. This can be the place where they will feel most safe and secure.

Living at home is the first choice for most of us: Couples almost always want to continue living together, and in some cultures multi-generational households are common. Families often find that close friends, neighbors, and family members can provide just enough help to make home care successful (see Asking for Help sidebar for more ideas on this topic). Although this informal caregiving is common, families eventually find that hiring occasional or ongoing help in the home becomes necessary. These in-home workers generally fall into two categories:

Home workers (sometimes called homemakers, caregivers, or personal care assistants). These versatile individuals will help with lighter chores such as housekeeping, laundry, meal preparation, and shopping. They may also help the person eat, bathe, dress, go to the bathroom, or manage incontinence. Many of these individuals now receive specialized training in dementia care, including learning how to engage the person in activities such as exercise, gardening, and simple chores. Part of the home worker's job may include watching an old movie with the person or going for a drive; families hire someone to provide care but also to provide stimulation and socialization.

Professional nursing staff. These more highly trained individuals may be hired to provide medications, injections, diabetes control, physical therapy, wound care, intravenous (IV) therapy, and occupational therapy. They will often monitor medication usage and may set up a weekly reminder box for medications to help the person accurately take prescriptions.

In-home workers can be hired privately or through a company. The latter option may be more expensive, but home care companies check employees' references, handle payroll and payroll taxes, provide staff training, and maintain appropriate insurance. Home care companies will also provide supervision and oversight, relieving you of the responsibility for managing all aspects of the employee–employer relationship.

If the person is low income, government financial assistance may be available for in-home help; in some states, this funding can even be used to pay a family member who is providing care. Check with your local Alzheimer's Association, Area Agency on Aging, senior service agency, or senior center for more information about paying for in-home care. Individuals who have purchased long-term care insurance will also find that these policies provide financial assistance.

Geriatric care managers. Another helpful resource can be *geriatric care managers*, who operate in many communities. These professionals (often nurses or social workers) are available to help you create a plan and identify resources, including benefits, for your family member. Many geriatric care managers provide bill-paying services and some have in-home workers available. Their services are generally provided on an hourly basis. They can be particularly helpful for long-distance family members, who can hire a local manager to oversee the care needs of the person more directly and be available for emergencies.

Hiring In-Home Help

If your preference is to hire someone privately, ask neighbors, friends, and family for recommendations. If you advertise on the Internet or in a newspaper/newsletter, do not put your address in the advertisement; doing this can create safety concerns. Conduct a thorough telephone interview to learn about the person's background and interest in home care. Trust your instincts. If the job candidate doesn't sound reliable, tell him or her that you have other telephone interviews to do and that you will call him or her if you want to do a future in-person interview.

It might be tempting to pay someone "under the table," but this is neither recommended nor legal. If the employee becomes disgruntled, is injured, or simply learns about his or her employment rights at a later date, the individual can make an expensive claim against you. If you are hiring your own worker, a payroll service can take care of tax reports and other responsibilities at a nominal cost.

Asking for Help

Care partners often hesitate to ask for help, yet friends and family often want to assist but don't know how. Here are some suggestions on how to ask friends and family for help:

- Be specific in requests: "Son, I would like you to come for Dad's birthday. Please make it a priority." A neighbor who wants to help might be asked to pick up some groceries occasionally.
- Do not assume family members should know your needs. Let them know what you need so they have a chance to help in their own way. Consider putting requests in writing to better communicate feelings and wishes, especially if you feel awkward asking for help.
- Recognize that family members are also coping with denial and other emotions about their loved one's illness. Give them time to cope.
- Recognize that some family members have the capacity to do more than others.
- Do not assume that requests for help will be a burden to family members. They often want to help and gain satisfaction from returning love and care.
- Try not to be overly critical or judgmental about others' attempts to provide help or support. Family members have different skills, different caregiving styles, and even different psychological constitutions.

When you meet or interview a candidate, see how he or she relates to the person. Ask the prospective worker to share any personal experiences of caring for an elderly relative or client. Is the candidate empathetic and loving? Does he or she seem to be knowledgeable and confident? Discuss your expectations. Always check references!

When looking at home-care options, many families today are choosing professional companies to find just the right worker and ensure that appropriate insurance, taxes, training, and supervision are present. Choose a reputable and established company and ask them to tell you how they train their employees to work with persons with dementia. How do they check employee references? Do they do criminal background checks? Sometimes the first person a company sends out just isn't a good match; don't give up hope. Even if it does take a few tries, you will soon find an effective and friendly worker to help you in the home.

With a private employee, create a simple contract or task list and have him or her review it before accepting your offer. This list should include work hours and the duties to be performed. Break the list down by household tasks (dust and vacuum, prepare lunch, wash dishes) and personal care (assist with tooth brushing, exercise/daily walk, assist with bath). Be aware that most workers will want a four-hour-per-day minimum. Most companies that offer in-home help will have their own "menu" of services and tasks; it can be helpful to choose from this list, which may include everything from bathing and toileting to doing laundry, cooking meals, or engaging in social activities.

Retaining in-home workers can be difficult. Be sure that you create an environment in which the employee feels valued. Sometimes the person with dementia and/or his care partner can be hard to please and difficult to work with. It is not unusual, in fact, for the person with Alzheimer's disease to "fire" (sometimes repeatedly) a great worker or reduce his or her hours to the point where the worker will not find it worthwhile to continue. The care partner sometimes has to intervene and ask the worker to keep coming. If your loved one does not live with you and you have arranged in-home care, be sure to keep in touch with the worker via phone, text message, or e-mail to reinforce that the work he or she is doing is valued and important.

One support group member told us that she used the knack of finesse with her parents who were reluctant to hire in-home help. After they had finally agreed to it, they had wanted to let the worker go just a week later despite the extended family's view that she was an exceptional employee. The daughter explained to her thrifty parents that the family had already paid her for the month and the money could not be refunded if they did not take advantage of her. The parents agreed to carry on, and by the end of the month they had adjusted to having in-home help, liked the worker, and wanted her to stay!

Do not forget to make use of the Life Story. Tell the worker about your loved one. Write a bullet card of key points for the worker to know (see page 115). When the worker knows your family member's likes, dislikes, routines, and preferences, everything will go better.

Above all, model good care and the Best Friends approach to your in-home workers. When they see you being kind and supportive of your loved one, you are setting an important example.

ADULT DAY CENTERS

Even when things are going well at home, we recommend that families consider adult day services. When we began our work in Alzheimer's disease in the early 1980s, most people thought of adult day centers strictly as respite services for care partners. It was quickly noticed, however, that the centers were doing much more than that—they were also helping the person with dementia with valuable socialization. Care partners reported that their loved ones seemed happier and exhibited fewer troublesome behaviors.

Dr. William R. Markesbery, founder of the University of Kentucky Alzheimer's Disease Research Center, was one of the leading dementia researchers in the world. After visiting the Best Friends Adult Day Center, he praised the outstanding activities and positive energy, saying, "This may be the treatment for dementia." Relationships and activities support happiness, reduce challenging behaviors, and create a therapeutic environment.

Through the years, many care partners have told us that their mother or father treats the staff and participants at the day center much better than he or she does family members. Perhaps this is because they are in a social setting, where old manners get put to work (that is, "It's not polite to be rude to strangers"), or it may just be the magic of friendship.

Adult day centers are usually open during standard working hours. They organize supervised activities for older adults and people with dementia. Some centers provide transportation. These centers may serve a mixed population that includes individuals with developmental disabilities, head injuries, or other special needs.

An adult day program is one of the best values in long-term care. Although daily costs vary, the maximum charge is usually much cheaper than a similar charge from a home care company or residential care facility. Many day centers are nonprofit and accept payment on a sliding fee scale. Day center care can be combined with in-home workers to maximize supervision and stretch your budget.

Respite is also critically important to the self-care of care partners. Day centers can provide an opportunity for you to play a round of golf, continue with employment, do projects around the house, visit friends, and take a break from the challenges of care. Some care partners tell us they use an adult day center care just to enjoy the luxury of being at home by themselves! This can be a time to get some filing done, take a nap, garden, or just put your feet up in a comfortable chair and read a good book. In addition, if your family member has had a busy day at the day center, he or she often comes home tired, which can ease your nighttime routine.

Encouraging Day Center Use

Many care partners are reluctant to use a day center. It is new to them. A typical argument is that Mother or Father "was never a joiner" and would not like the program or would be somehow embarrassed by it. From our experience, it is true that the person with dementia will almost never initially embrace the idea of day care. He or she will need to be encouraged by the family. Here are some tips for encouraging a reluctant loved one to use day center care:

- Cast it as a social club or outing that will keep the person active.
- Get a physician to "prescribe" day center use two or three times a week for eight weeks.
- Go with the person the first time or two and have lunch or coffee together at the center.
- Encourage the person to be a "volunteer" at the center.

Often, after the person falls into a routine, the day center becomes a source of friendship, happiness, and physical and mental stimulation. Day centers are good for you and good for the person with dementia. In addition, day centers are often activity rich. In fact, if you are struggling to find things to do at home on the weekends or evenings, spend some time at the day program and borrow some of their ideas.

Alzheimer's Cafés

Alzheimer's cafés are places where persons with dementia and their families can come for some social activity, support, and refreshments. The concept started in the Netherlands in 1997 as a hybrid between a day center and support group. They are springing up around the world and proving popular. A British group, Alzheimer Café UK, offers a website featuring information about the history of the concept and a helpful how-to fact sheet (www.alzheimercafe.co.uk). In the United States, a number of the local chapters of the Alzheimer's Association host Alzheimer's cafés. Dr. Deborah Danner of the University of Kentucky Alzheimer's Disease Research Center hosts a monthly café and says: "The meeting has proved popular with persons with dementia and their families. Sometimes over twenty are present and it's amazing how much conversation and fun goes on. You wouldn't know that half the people present have dementia!"

When Parents Refuse Their Children's Help

When one person in a couple is diagnosed with Alzheimer's disease or other dementia, it can prove very traumatic. Your parents may want to try to handle it all by themselves. Here are some ways to be an effective adult-child care partner:

- Call or visit often; try to be helpful in ways that are acceptable (errands, driving them places, or yard work, for example).
- Pick your battles! The way the caregiving parent used to keep the house and yard, or even the way he or she used to dress, may not be important now. He or she may have different priorities.
- Don't become the "bad guy" through constant criticism or nagging or by continuing to give unsolicited suggestions.
- Be patient. Almost always, the caregiving parent will eventually reach out for help from adult children if you continue to be supportive and understanding.

RESIDENTIAL CARE

Most family care partners think that placement in an assisted living community, special dementia care unit, or skilled nursing facility is a last resort. Family concerns about making a placement include:

- Guilt about their decision.
- Not knowing how to make the transition out of the home happen.
- Fear that their loved one will not be happy, will get hurt, will wander off, or otherwise not make a successful transition into the facility.

- Fear that if the placement does not work out, the person may have to return home or move again.

The Martyrdom Trap

When a care partner complains about his or her job while at the same time refusing all offers of help, he or she has fallen into the martyrdom trap. It happens frequently, in part because of the intensity of the caregiving role and the fact that care partners become tired, begin to exercise poor judgment, and sometimes fall into denial. Being a martyr—giving up your life for someone else or some cause—is only a short-term strategy at best. You want to be there for the long run—for the person in your care, for your friends and family, and for yourself. Practice saying "yes" instead of "no."

While these feelings and concerns are very real, the transition into residential care often goes surprisingly well and proves to be a good thing for the person and his or her family. A residential care community can, for example, support better physical care (such as more frequent bathing), provide more activities, offer a more regular routine, and ensure a more nutritious and varied menu. The person with dementia may also benefit from and enjoy the activity programs and socialization that accompany group living.

The promise to "always keep Mother at home" might have been made with the best of intentions and hopes, but sometimes the care partner him- or herself is in frail health. (See "Substituted Judgment" sidebar on page 237 for more on the topic of promises.) Care at home may simply become too demanding.

We view it as a positive trend that specialized dementia care programs have become more common. Many are doing a good job with innovative and interesting activities and staff who are specifically trained in dementia care. Well ahead of the time you might make a move, visit several programs in your community to identify the best one(s); this is much better than making a decision under duress. Talk to the program director. Does he or she seem knowledgeable and inspire confidence? Look at the activity program; is it contemporary and interesting or does it default to Bingo and crafts? Is the environment warm and inviting, clean, and well lit? Does it evoke feelings of home? Do staff members know and use the residents' life stories? Does the team have the training and skill to handle behavioral issues if and when they arise? For more advice on choosing a residential care program and making the move, see the book *Moving a Relative with Memory Loss: A Family Caregiver's Guide* by Laurie White and Beth Spencer, an excellent guide listed in the Recommended Readings section.

Residential care falls into two major categories: assisted living and skilled nursing facilities.

What Is the Ombudsman Program?

Available throughout the United States, the long-term care ombudsman program has staff and volunteers who serve as advocates for individuals in assisted living and skilled residential care programs. Ombudsman offices also maintain lists of licensing violations against area facilities. Before making a placement or beginning your search, visit or call your ombudsman office (listed in the telephone book under "Ombudsman" or "Long-term Care Ombudsman"). They can be a friend to the family considering placement, can provide an up-to-date list of facilities (usually with prices), and provide advice about the search process.

Once your loved one is placed in residential care, the ombudsman office can continue to help by mediating any complaints or concerns that might arise that you are unable to resolve directly with the facility's administration. The ombudsman program can also be helpful if you believe your loved one is being evicted from a facility without good reason.

Assisted Living

Assisted living has been a growth industry in the last decade. Across the country communities are being built to provide a caring home that can provide necessary help to our growing numbers of elders. Many of these communities feature dementia care neighborhoods; some are entirely for persons with dementia. Assisted living communities are known by many names, depending on the state in which you live. Some of these include residential care, personal care, adult congregate care, and board-and-home care. Common to all these terms, however, is the understanding that an assisted living setting is a group residential setting that provides or coordinates meals and personal services, 24-hour supervision and assistance (scheduled and unscheduled), activities, and health-related services. Monthly prices for dementia care in assisted living vary across the country but in 2012 they averaged between $5,000 and $6,000 per month.

Assisted living communities house as few as a handful of residents up to hundreds of residents. Most assisted living programs are for privately paying individuals, although some do accept lower-income individuals through various government programs. Because most people with dementia, through much of their illness, primarily need supervision and assistance with everyday activities and personal care rather than health care from medically trained professionals, assisted living is generally the best level of residential care for them.

Some assisted living communities are quite lavish and feature lovely great rooms, country kitchens, and beautiful gardens. Others are much more modest. As you look for an assisted living community, keep in mind that the most important factor is the staff and the program. Having a beautiful space is a plus, but it doesn't compensate for a lethargic or untrained staff and boring or limited activities. Kay Kallander, Senior Vice President for Strategic Planning for American Baptist Homes of the West says it best: "When looking for staff, hire for the heart, train for the task." The best assisted living programs have staff motivated by friendship and love for persons with dementia.

Skilled Nursing Communities

Skilled nursing communities provide twenty-four-hour nursing care, and their licenses and staffing allow them to accept individuals with greater medical and care needs. This level is expensive if you are paying privately—sometimes $100,000 a year or more. Medicare does pay for skilled nursing care, but it only covers short-term placements and is generally only for rehabilitation services after a hospitalization. If the person is eligible for Medicaid, funding is available for skilled nursing care over a long-term basis. Although state regulations vary, persons with dementia generally are appropriate for this level of care if they have medical needs that require greater nursing supervision. Examples include needing oxygen or catheters, not being ambulatory, or having swallowing and eating difficulties. In some cases persons with dementia who need extraordinary help with personal care (for example, requiring two staff members to help in the shower) or who have ongoing falls may need to be at this level of care.

Sadly, many of these skilled nursing communities have shared and cramped rooms, long corridors, and an institutional environment that resembles a hospital more than a home. Despite these detractions, staff members at this demanding level of care usually have great heart and dedication.

Elders Living Alone

One growing trend is that of single elders living at home alone. If these individuals develop dementia, the home can become a very unsafe place. The person can accidentally start a fire, fall and not be found for hours or days, become malnourished, fail to take medications properly, or wander off.

If you have a friend or family member living alone, or are concerned about a frail older couple, often the best approach is to stay in touch, avoid being demanding or critical, and quietly investigate various services and programs. You can also ask neighbors or nearby friends to be "good Samaritans" and keep an eye on things or drop by occasionally. Many communities have outreach, or "friendly visiting" programs, for these individuals so that they do not become isolated and unsafe. However, if the person refuses help (for example, doesn't accept a Meals on Wheels type of service and claims to be eating well), and he or she is still legally competent, then there is not much you can do legally to force the issue.

If a person is at risk to him- or herself or others (for example, as in the above paragraph becoming dangerously malnourished versus just not eating well), the Adult Protective Services (APS) program can spring into action. Many professionals are, in fact, "mandated reporters" and must call APS if they suspect elder abuse or neglect. Other actions might include appointing a public guardian or getting a friend or family member to file for a conservatorship to manage the person's legal and/or health affairs.

CONTINUING CARE RETIREMENT COMMUNITIES (CCRC)

It is a growing trend to have a variety of senior services all on one campus. The result is the continuing care retirement community (CCRC). These campuses usually include apartments and houses for independent seniors, assisted living, memory care, and skilled nursing. Some CCRCs also have adult day programs and in-home support available. Many of these communities are nonprofit and some are faith based. Several financial options may exist for moving into a CCRC but most require some kind of buy-in, which in turn guarantees lifetime housing and increased levels of care as needs change. Most have dementia care programs for their residents. The dementia programs give first priority to current residents, but many do have openings from time to time and may be a good option to consider.

Evaluating the Setting

A quality dementia-specific care program should have the following:

- **A good record with its licensing agency:** Check with your local long-term care ombudsman office to review any complaints or health citations. Do the complaints suggest an ongoing pattern of poor care or are they isolated events? What has been the facility's response to complaints? Very few facilities are complaint free, but you want to choose one that has a good track record overall and that is held in high regard by regulators and/or ombudsman programs.
- **A written philosophy of care:** Administrators of special care programs should be able to describe their care goals to potential residents and families. They should be able to explain why they are special.
- **Intensive staffing ratios:** Because dementia care demands superior supervision, a special care program should have higher staff-to-resident ratios.
- **Thoughtful care planning:** Special care programs should place extra emphasis on care planning, involving an interdisciplinary team to set appropriate goals and monitor each resident's program.
- **An emphasis on staff training:** Special care programs should offer intensive and extensive training to their staff members. Ask the administrator how the staff is trained. Good programs supplement in-house training with guest speakers and opportunities for staff members to attend workshops and conferences. Does the community have a relationship with the local Alzheimer's Association or other local dementia support organization?
- **A dementia-friendly physical environment:** The best special care units have architectural design elements that are dementia-

friendly. These elements might include wandering paths, raised garden beds, open kitchens, seating areas to encourage conversation and activity, secure perimeters, good lighting, and soothing colors. It is important to note, however, that the best architectural design will fail if staff do not have knack; a good program could be held in a barn with the right staff.

These factors describe an ideal situation. In the real world, you may or may not live in a community with lots of choices. Those people with limited financial assets or income are likely to have fewer choices. Some communities have plenty of openings; others have waiting lists.

Substituted Judgment

Many family members tell us how they promised their dad (or other relative) that they would always keep Mom at home. Or families have made the promise directly to the person, saying he or she could always stay at home.

We recognize that these promises carry great significance for families. It is hard to entertain the idea of breaking this promise. We would argue, however, that there are times when families need to consider doing just that.

Sometimes a person simply is not safe at home. He or she wanders, overflows the bathtub, or starts fires on the stove. Other times, the person's isolation becomes profound and he or she becomes depressed. If living alone, the person's health and personal care may suffer, particularly if the person refuses in-home help.

Families suffer over this situation, siblings often argue, and the stress and worry grow.

How can a family deal with the tough reality of the situation and weigh this against a promise? The concept of *substituted judgment* may help.

Substituted judgment is the idea in ethics that one can make a decision for someone else if he or she is impaired. We do this by imagining what the person would say if he or she was able to weigh in on the topic.

Let's say you are in this dilemma and have promised your mother she can always stay home. Now she is becoming a danger to herself. Perhaps she is being hoodwinked by door-to-door salespeople and wandering at night. Pose the question: If I could roll back the clock and ask Mother, what would she want me to do in this circumstance? Nine times out of ten, families begin to realize that Mother would have wanted you to protect her and her finances by acting to change the situation. Nine times out of ten, Mother would have wanted you to take care of yourself and not let her care overwhelm the family.

Substituted judgment can help us look at a caregiving situation with fresh eyes and make the best decision for our family member and for ourselves.

MAKING THE MOVE FROM HOME

It is a day almost every family dreads: the day you take Mom or Dad, or your spouse or partner, to a facility. Families vary in their attitudes about whether to discuss the situation ahead of time. It is always advisable to discuss the move with the person when possible. It can be framed in many ways, including "doctor's orders" or a "temporary vacation or stay" or even just as a measure to take because the care partner is ailing. But often, a person with dementia is so forgetful and has such poor judgment that talking about this move ahead of time will have no payoff; it would just alarm and upset the person.

In this case, family members have taken their loved ones for a drive, have come to "visit" the residential community, and have broken the news to them at that point. Staff can work with families ahead of time to decorate the room with some of the person's belongings, which can help the person adapt more quickly to a change in living arrangements.

How to Visit

Friends and family often find it difficult or depressing to visit their loved one in residential care, particularly as their loved one's dementia worsens. What do you talk about? What do you do? Does the person really know if you are there?

It is important to maintain a presence at your loved one's residential home. First, you want to monitor the care he or she is getting. In general, shorter, more frequent visits are recommended if you find it hard to visit at length. Second, you want to give the person emotional support and help with any other aspects of care that need attention. If you can't visit on a regular basis, ask for help from friends and family. If your loved one belonged to a certain social club or fraternity, ask the members to set up a visiting schedule.

Visits do not have to be elaborate. Bring along your checkbook to balance in the person's room, read some magazines, or do some shopping by catalog. It's your physical presence that may mean the most to the person. Bring in baked goods to share with your loved one, other residents, and staff. Arrive armed with the latest family photographs.

Finally, ask to be part of the facility's regular care management conferences so you can sit in on care meetings that concern your loved one.

Once a placement is made, it always takes time for the person to adjust. We have seen many different outcomes. Sometimes the person you least expect to accept the placement thrives. Other times the person remains angry and upset. The knack of patience and empathy is important here. Making an adjustment like this would be hard on any of us. Hopefully, a caring staff, good food, creative activities, and your ongoing presence as a care partner will help make the placement successful. Your own positive attitude will also provide reassurance. Even though guilt, loss, and other negative feelings are common and understandable in this situation, do your best to avoid negativity around the person. This doesn't mean denying your own feelings; give yourself time to get in touch with and accept the emotions raised by this change in your family life. Be reassured that most of these transitions are successful and the person benefits from good personal care and life-affirming activities. Sometimes residential programs suggest that family members not visit for two or more weeks to let the person adjust. Although this may be good advice in some circumstances, in most cases the person will benefit from supportive visits and reassurance from loved ones during his or her adjustment to a new home.

Getting the Best Care from a Residential Care Community

Once a placement has been made, work to make sure your relationship with staff members is productive. Many staff members have complained to us that family members are overly critical, sometimes even hostile. While you may have legitimate concerns, burning bridges or developing a reputation as a "challenging family member" almost never benefits your loved one. Here are some ideas for building a more positive relationship with the staff:

- **Be part of the team.** Families can enhance the quality of care by helping out at meals now and then and doing one-to-one activities.
- **Pick your issues.** If your mother is in pajamas late one morning, perhaps she wanted it that way or perhaps the staff fell behind. This is not as important as being timely with medications or nutrition.
- **Recognize that it's a dementia program.** Don't sweat the small stuff such as socks being misplaced or someone else wearing your mother's bathrobe. Items move around in a community filled with individuals with memory loss.
- **Model behavior for the staff.** If you want them to approach your mother in a certain way or to talk about a favorite subject, let staff hear you do the same. For example, if you know your mother loves going out on to the patio, take her out there and then let the staff know that you and your mother have enjoyed the sunshine and roses.

When you have a concern or complaint, voice it. Some families hesitate to do this out of fear of retribution. Well-run and ethical communities will welcome your feedback and do their best to address your concerns. Two tips will help this go better:

1. Be sure to address your concern to the right staff member. A nursing assistant on the night shift may not be the person to complain to about something that happened during the day,

and he or she might not have the authority to follow up on your concern.

2. Adopt an old management trick and be sure to couch your complaints with what you think is going well (and hopefully some things will be going well). Rightly or wrongly, if the staff sees you as a chronic complainer, they will begin to avoid you or will not hear your words.

Families are sometimes dissatisfied with a residential program and wonder if it will be too disruptive to move their family member. The answer is complex and varies by situation. Change is hard for persons with dementia, but it is also important for them to be in a good program. If you feel a program has not kept its promises, consider a move to a competitor. Persons with dementia can be surprisingly resilient and will respond positively to a move when the new staff and environment are more positive. No program is perfect, so weigh your decision carefully if you are thinking about a change. You do have the right to expect excellence for your money.

FEELING GOOD ABOUT YOUR PLACEMENT DECISION

Doctors, family members, friends, and even neighbors will offer well-intended advice such as, "You should place him when he no longer knows you." "You should place her when she becomes incontinent." "You should place him when he doesn't sleep through the night." "You have no choice. You must place her now." It is important to follow your own instincts and take care of your own needs. We all have differing skill levels, coping mechanisms, values, personalities, and resources that may play a role in making a decision to keep someone at home or move them into a care setting. Bear in mind that responsibilities don't end at placement, either; care partners often still have responsibilities for buying supplies, providing medications, attending care planning meetings, and taking the person to medical appointments.

We knew one care partner who masterfully tackled the toughest aspects of care for her husband, handling many difficult personal care choices, dressing and bathing him, taking him to a day center, and designing activities for him. Her "breaking point" came when he began to have trouble climbing the stairs to their second-floor bedroom. When the doctor suggested putting a hospital bed downstairs in her formal dining room, she decided it was something she could never do—disturb her cherished formal dining room and the symbolic structure in her life it represented. She then made a placement. This is an unusual example, but it shows that the decision to make a placement is based on many variables, some of them surprising. There is no simple formula.

Several things are important for you to consider when deciding on a placement in residential care:

- **Rethink past promises.** What is most important now is the quality of life for the person and for you.
- **Consider the benefits of placement to the person.** Many persons thrive, eat better, receive expert personal care, and come out of isolation in a residential setting.

- **Take advantage of local resources for help with the decision.** Many communities have nonprofit agencies that will guide you through the placement process.
- **Identify potential residential care programs early.** Many of the best places have waiting lists. If you wait until a crisis hits, you may find your options very limited.
- **Investigate social programs that might help**. The Veterans' Administration is a good resource for many. Medicaid does cover skilled care. A good elder-law attorney can sometimes help preserve assets and plan for the future.

END-OF-LIFE CARE

Many hospice programs are finding that an increasing percentage of their clients have dementia. They have acquired the experience and skills to support the person and his or her family in the final stages of this disease.

Hospice programs provide medical and social support along with bereavement counseling. When a person qualifies for hospice, that program becomes the care manager for everything from managing medications to arranging for staff to come and help give a bath or shower. Medicare will cover the cost of hospice services.

It is important to look ahead to end-of-life issues. Have conversations with the person (when possible) and his or her family about personal philosophies and goals. Hopefully the person has created an advanced directive or communicated his or her wishes relating to end-of-life care. When a person reaches late-stage dementia, many families work with their physician and pharmacist to limit medications to the most essential ones and/or the ones that support comfort. Families may also choose not to aggressively treat conditions such as pneumonia or heart failure, believing that quality of life trumps the "quantity" of life. Most of us want to live a long, *good* life, not just a long life.

CONCLUSION

Many families consider the use of community services as a defeat or a negative reflection on their own caregiving skills. The opposite is true: Using community-based services tells others that you are a resourceful and effective care partner and, in fact, gives you more options. Using a day center or hiring in-home help also generally allows you to care for the person with dementia at home longer.

If the time comes when a residential care placement is needed, it is important to know that caregiving does not end here, it just changes. Often the care partner who has been giving the bath, helping the person get dressed, fixing the meals, and helping the person out of a chair on a continual basis finds a tremendous weight lifted when others take over these tasks. Instead of struggling in the shower, you can now go visit the person and take a walk, have a meal, or spend some quality time together.

More and more long-term care programs are adopting the Best Friends model as their own philosophy of care. In these communities, they teach staff how to be Best Friends care partners by encouraging them to learn as much as possible about your loved one, enjoy creative activities, and provide the person with good care. They become partners in helping your loved one lead a dignified life.

Best Friends Pointers

- Don't wait to use services. In-home help can give you respite, provide support with personal care, and provide your family member with valuable socialization.
- Activity-rich adult day centers are particularly valuable services.
- Many residential care communities have dementia-specific programs with environments that are caring, engaging, and safe and secure for your family member.
- Even if you don't think you will use residential care, it can be smart to study the local market, visit communities, and even get on waiting lists.
- Ask family members and friends for help when you need it. Many will rise to the occasion and be supportive if you just tell them what you need.

IV

LIVING WITH DIGNITY

11

SELF-CARE

Being Your Own Best Friend

On commercial airlines, flight attendants tell you that if the emergency oxygen masks need to be used, you should put on your own oxygen mask first before attending to a child or companion. The point is, if you do not take care of yourself first, you will not be in a position to help others. This is especially important in dementia care because the care partner's journey can be a long one.

As a care partner, it is essential to be your own Best Friend for your own sake. Only then can you provide good-quality care to your loved one who needs it. The Best Friends approach can help you gain more satisfaction from your care of an individual with dementia, improve his or her quality of life, and nurture connections among you and your family members.

This journey of acceptance and growth is beautifully described in a series of diary entries and Christmas letters written by Jo Riley, husband to Rebecca Riley, which you can read at the end of this chapter. You have already learned something about Rebecca's experience as a younger person diagnosed with Alzheimer's disease, but now you can also see this experience from the perspective of her Best Friend and care partner.

Also, for the person with Alzheimer's disease or other dementia, being your own Best Friend starts with using your strengths for as long as possible and surrounding yourself with Best Friends. It may also involve adopting a particular philosophy, such as Rebecca Riley's decision to live one day at a time, Beverly Wheeler's intention to teach others, Dicy Jenkins's steadfast belief in a higher power, Dorothy Troxel's ability to enjoy a fun tea party with friends, or Jerry Ruttenberg's continuing reliance on his sense of humor. Details from the Alzheimer's experience of each of these individuals have been shared throughout this book; you can learn more from their "Biographies" at the end of the book.

WAYS TO TAKE CARE OF YOUR OWN NEEDS

Following is a list of things you can do to help take care of yourself. Yet, just as every person with dementia is different, every family's situation is different. We hope that one or more of these ideas will be helpful to you.

Set Realistic Expectations

Because you care about your loved ones, you can easily lose sight of how much you can realistically give. Ask the following questions: What is the state of my health? How much of the physical care can I reasonably provide, if any? How much time can I spend on caregiving (away from employment or other family obligations)? What kind of family support do I have? How much money can I spend on caring for my loved one without jeopardizing my family's financial well-being?

Review Your Living Situation

Step back from the journey to assess your living situation. Are you close to services or way out in a rural area? Is there a ground-floor bedroom and accessible bathroom? Is the house free from tripping hazards such as electrical cords? Is the lighting adequate?

Some families opt to have their loved one move into residential care or move closer to children. Try not to rush into hasty decisions. In-home care or support from a good day center can also be options. Be sure to give yourself some time after a diagnosis to carefully consider your options.

Use Services Early and Often

The previous chapter offered a helpful discussion of available services. Using support services early and often benefits you by connecting you to well-informed and supportive professionals who can offer not only education but important respite.

Rebecca and Jo Riley looked for a support group for both of them, agreed to utilize an adult day center, and eventually traveled the journey into residential care. Jo involved Rebecca in these decisions as much as possible. Each of these programs was a lifeline for them, where they could meet others going through the same experience. Most of the services also provide persons like Rebecca with needed socialization.

Find a Confidante

A trusted friend or counselor can make all the difference. You need someone to talk things over with, someone who will be nonjudgmental, respect confidentiality, and be understanding of your needs. A good counselor can help you or your family problem-solve, vent frustration, communicate more effectively, and make important decisions. To find a counselor, ask friends or colleagues, contact your local Alzheimer's Association or Society, or check with your local Area Agency on Aging or senior center.

Jo turned to his children often to share his feelings. All through his diary he speaks about being close to them. Their acceptance and support was a wonderful gift to Jo and Rebecca.

Sometimes all it takes is one friend or family member to provide a shoulder to cry on or to be a good listener.

Practice Assertiveness

Often, it is difficult to express your feelings and needs. When stress or fatigue increases, it can be even harder. Practice assertiveness, and do not be afraid to speak up to family members and friends about your feelings and needs. It is okay to admit that you are confused or need more information and help. See page 223, Asking for Help, for a review of key ideas on this topic.

> *Jo tells this story in his diary: "We had an interview with a social worker and a nurse about a support group for Rebecca. They did not talk directly to Rebecca but always asked me and directed the conversation toward me. That made Rebecca feel left out. When I called it to their attention they were surprised and shocked."*

Jo's assertiveness helped the professionals learn to be more empathetic and sensitive to Rebecca. Rather than walking away in anger, he provided feedback that helped preserve the relationship with the social worker and nurse who did have valuable information to share.

Develop Strategies for Handling Unhelpful Advice

Advice from a trusted friend or professional can be helpful, but care partners sometimes find themselves deluged with unsolicited suggestions. Friends and family mean well but sometimes their suggestions or comments, such as "Put him in a nursing home" or "She doesn't seem that bad to me," can create more stress. Helpful advice is a gift, but if the advice is not helpful or if it seems critical, develop a few stock responses such as "Thanks for your input" or "Thanks for your concern."

Maintain Contact with the Outside World

Care partners who devote all of their energy toward their loved one can inadvertently shut out friends and family. Often, care partners must cut back on commitments and social activities, but balance is important. Make at least one call each week to a friend you have been too busy to see or talk to. You can also make new friends through support groups, introductions to families at day centers, or other programs that help families coping with dementia.

Jo kept working as a pastor well into Rebecca's illness. After she died, he attended classes at the University of Kentucky.

Doing this helped Jo maintain his self-esteem and confidence, and kept him engaged with friends and other professionals.

Simplify Your Life

When your mother or spouse has a closet full of clothes and a collection of 200 ceramic bunnies you can often feel overwhelmed by all the things in the house. Too many clothes in the closet, for example, can make it harder to get the person dressed and harder to find things. Many care partners have taken this opportunity to discreetly dispose of "white elephants" and get down to the basics. Simplicity makes your daily routine easier and reduces stress.

Jo and Rebecca were wise to admit that their house was becoming too difficult to manage. They chose to dispose of much of their "stuff" and move to an apartment in a retirement center.

Fulfill Creative Impulses

Many care partners find that creative expression can be a positive way to cope with dementia. Care partners have written (poems, plays, novels, even an opera), produced films, journaled, and painted about their experiences. Creative expressions can help you channel your anger and despair into more positive outlets.

After Rebecca moved into assisted living, Jo was able to take a week off to help others: "I spent a week in Florida as a volunteer for Habitat for Humanity." Participating in the creative process of designing and building a new home for others allowed him to stay connected to his long-standing interest in community engagement.

Building something with his hands that had a beginning, middle, and end was satisfying to Jo and fulfilled him at many levels, including a need to be creative.

Listen to Your Body

People providing care to individuals with dementia are at greater risk for premature disability and death than others of similar age who are not providing care. This is the result of numerous factors, notably the stress that comes from the tasks of caregiving. Make a concerted effort to eat properly, exercise, and pamper yourself. Consider getting regular massages or practicing meditation, among other rewards.

Be Good to Yourself

Zealously carve out time for yourself and try to maintain special activities, hobbies, friendships, or other things that give pleasure. You should also give yourself presents whenever possible, such as an afternoon to go fishing or fresh flowers from the local farmers' market.

Jo found it satisfying to spend time at his favorite place: "We went to our cottage on Crystal Lake. We had all the family there and had a good time."

Some professionals might have felt that going on a vacation would be "too much" for Rebecca. On the contrary, she enjoyed being in an old, familiar place that was beautiful, calm, and relaxing.

Plan Ahead

Because the progression of Alzheimer's disease and other dementia is often slow, families usually have time to plan ahead. Consider, for example, the possibility that the other person might outlive you. Without a workable plan for this circumstance, a family's financial affairs and care plan for the person can be disrupted.

Forgive Others and Yourself

Alzheimer's disease finds people at their best and at their worst. When friends or family say or do the wrong thing, it is valuable to look at the underlying motive. That motive may be love and concern, even if what is said or done is not helpful. It is also true that the best care partners are often hardest on themselves. Give yourself permission to make mistakes, to have bad days, and to think angry, even shameful, thoughts. Even the closest friends have their ups and downs.

Write Down Your Caregiving Experiences

Many care partners, like Jo Riley, find that keeping a diary or writing notes about the experience can be helpful. If you jot down patterns of behavior, a diary can even become a problem-solving tool. It can provide a safe place to write about stresses, strains, and feelings; you can "vent" and say things you cannot say in public.

Fulfill Your Own Spiritual Needs

When bad news hits, many of us turn to our religious traditions or other spiritual pathways (like the arts and time spent in nature) to help make sense of the news. Traveling these paths can help you cope and give you strength. No matter how tough things are, care partners who take time to find the spiritual in themselves and who reach out to friends and family and their faith communities will experience more success.

> *Jo remained close to his faith community. His spirit was also enhanced by his love of nature: "Our summer was filled by drinking in beautiful sunsets, the blue skies, the sand dunes, the birds, and enjoying our many friends in Michigan."*

Jo's spirit was touched by his religious faith as well as the magnificence of Mother Nature.

Maintain a Sense of Humor

The art of providing good care involves maintaining a sense of humor and striving to lighten up about life's challenges. Watching a classic comedy movie or program on television, sharing a funny story at a support group meeting, or simply laughing with the person can help inoculate you against the stress and strain of caregiving.

WHEN EVERYTHING IS GOING WRONG

Even people who practice the Best Friends approach will find the challenges of caregiving overwhelming at times. Alzheimer's disease can pose tremendous challenges to the most skilled care partner.

For example, if the person has an undetected infection or is in pain, behaviors can throw a well-planned activity into chaos. Sometimes care partners get into such a slump (perhaps because of depression, fatigue, frail health) that they find it hard to take action. Their judgment can become clouded. Family dynamics can work for or against the care partner. In some cases, the care of the person is not the major challenge, but handling family disagreements and conflicts are.

One of the most important ways to be one's own Best Friend is to take advantage of respite care opportunities. Our first choice is an adult day center. However, informal respite opportunities, such as saying yes to a friend or family member who offers to come and help for an afternoon, are also good options.

The following list of ideas of how to cope when everything seems to be going wrong has come from members of support groups. Some ideas are serious, others a little outrageous, but they are all examples of "stress busters" that help us learn to be our own Best Friends:

- Take a day off and do whatever you want.
- Wait until a train is passing, then go outside and scream as loud as you can.
- Call a friend to come over to be with you.
- Read a joke book.
- Hug a friend.
- Call your minister/priest/rabbi to share your feelings.
- Buy a new outfit.
- Eat chocolate, chocolate, chocolate.
- Take a long walk in nature.
- Order a pizza, and eat it all.

- Spend a weekend at a retreat center.
- Be humble enough to accept help and support.
- Have a good, therapeutic cry!

CONCLUSION

The Best Friends approach suggests that the caregiving experience is like one door closing and another opening. One care partner jotted down the following words when thinking about his future: *new friends and relationships, travel, new hobbies, laughter, tears, healing, and pride in a job well done.* Being one's own Best Friend maximizes quality of life during the sometimes arduous tasks of caregiving. Even more important, it positions one for a life after Alzheimer's disease or other dementia.

It is important for you to consider where you want to be in life in one year, three years, or ten years. Think about what relationships you want to have with your family and friends. What do you want to be able to say about your time as a care partner? The Best Friends approach is a life raft being thrown to you—a chance to redirect disappointment, anger, and pain, and instead find moments of joy in day-to-day caregiving. We ask you to be open to change. The Best Friends approach cannot take away a diagnosis of Alzheimer's disease or other dementia, but it can improve quality of life for you and your loved one.

Best Friends Pointers

- Don't wait and wait to use services or fall into martyrdom. Services can be good for the person and good for you.
- Lighten up on life. Decide what is important and what is not that important at this time in your life.
- Keep in touch with friends and family and continue as many of your everyday activities as possible.
- Take one day at a time.
- Forgive yourself for mistakes and strive to make tomorrow a better day.

THE POWER OF A DIARY: REBECCA AND JO RILEY

The following pages contain excerpts from Jo Riley's writings from the date of the diagnosis of his wife, Rebecca, in 1984 through 1999. We find his words valuable because they demonstrate that one can be a good and dedicated caregiver while being intentional about acting as one's own Best Friend. Except for minor editing for clarity, the words are Jo's.

July 30, 1984: When we went to see our neurologist after all the tests were in, he just very quietly said that Rebecca had Alzheimer's disease. We were devastated! We knew something was wrong and were hoping that it would be a brain tumor or something else. . . . We left Barnes Hospital and drove toward Centralia, Illinois, . . . and had lunch. It was a sober lunch and a very quiet one. We resolved that we were going to make the best of it and live one day at a time.

When we learned of her diagnosis, I recalled that Rebecca began having trouble about a year and a half ago pronouncing some words. She was an excellent reader and a fast reader. She stumbled over some of these words, and I didn't think anything about it. I recall now that was the first sign of trouble.

November 1984: We had an interview with a nurse and a social worker about a support group for Rebecca. They did not talk directly to Rebecca, but always asked me and directed the conversation toward me. This made Rebecca feel left out. When I called it to their attention, they were surprised and shocked. I think this is the first time that I had felt that social workers and nurses and doctors were thinking only of the families, they are not thinking of the patient. We learned there was a support group for caregivers but none for the patient.

Spring 1985: We planned our move to retire in Kentucky. I have been noticing that Rebecca is still having trouble reading and that she is having some trouble in writing. She is constantly referring to the dictionary and having trouble finding words. Our children have been fully supportive and want us to come by and see them.

June 1985: We went to Crystal Lake in Northern Michigan. We had a summer that was filled with visits. Our families knew of her condition, but Rebecca was beginning to feel left out. I think she wanted to talk to them about her illness but they were afraid to. This is another example of the loneliness that crept into her.

January 1986: We went to Hopkinsville, Kentucky, for an interim ministry. While we've been in Hopkinsville, I've noticed some things. She has always been an outgoing person, speaking and teaching. I've noticed that she is more withdrawn; she's scared of people because she can't remember names. She's writing names down every place but has trouble remembering them. Her reading may be a little worse, but her writing is still good and legible. She has a hard time getting out the words she wants.

The trouble with Alzheimer's disease is when people know someone has it they immediately shy away from the person. Rebecca knows this as a nurse. She sees it now that she has Alzheimer's and it is a very depressing state. We as a people do not know how to treat people who are sick. They want to talk about it, but we are afraid to talk about it. The dictionary is now her constant companion. We need something for Rebecca. We feel that there is a need for a support group for the patient.

Summer 1986: We went to our cottage at Crystal Lake. We had all the family there, and it was a good time. I noticed that it takes Rebecca longer to plan and execute the plan. One thing that I have noticed is that Rebecca has talked more in the past year about getting a dog or pet. She has empathy for people and animals. She has commented about the butterflies; while driving, she doesn't want to kill one or an animal. She loves birds and loves to watch them. I've noticed that she wants me with her more than ever. I guess she wants reassurance.

October 1986: Rebecca is carrying on as usual. She's cooking, she's doing her needlepoint, she's singing in a church choir, and she is going with me whenever I go out of town. Sometimes I notice she doesn't want to talk, and other times she enters into conversation.

She is carrying the checkbook and is doing a very good job writing a check. She said she is afraid of writing a check, but so far she has been very accurate. I think in writing the check she gets confused when having to write out the words on the check. She gets stopped on the spelling of "hundred" or whatever the figure is. She wrote all our thank you's and kept them up to date. Thus far we know of no medicine, no treatment, or no cure. We're living one day at a time.

CHRISTMAS SALUTATIONS

The following are the Rileys' Christmas letters, which further chronicle Rebecca's and Jo's experiences with Alzheimer's disease.

1987: At Christmas, our daughter Joetta and her husband Bill called us to say that they wanted to bring two friends with them. We said OK. It turned out to be two dogs. When they left, we were the proud owners of "Corky," a Chinese Shih Tzu. He thinks that he is a person and is always at our feet.

Christmas is the spirit of love, which God has gratefully given to each of us and we extend to you. At Christmas time, the angels sang of peace and goodwill, which is translated, "Love to you."

—Rebecca and Jo

1988: Jo served as interim minister for two months at Woodmount Christian Church in Nashville. It was a great experience working with the staff in this large metropolitan church. The byproduct was visiting many historical sites around Nashville.

After three weeks home in Lexington, we were off to the USSR for a pilgrimage to the Russian Orthodox Church, which celebrated their 1,000th year.

Rebecca had a big time in May when her family had a family reunion.

Christmas is the spirit of love, which God has gratefully given to each of us and we extend to you our love.

—Rebecca and Jo

1989: We got back home from the lake. Our summer was filled by drinking in beautiful sunsets, the blue skies, the sand dune, the birds, and enjoying the many friends in Michigan. We are enjoying our retirement with Corky, who requires a walk twice a day. May the love of Christmas be yours and warm your hearts and fill your life with Love.

—Rebecca and Jo

1990: The big news of 1990 for the Rileys was our move. In February we decided to move to Richmond Place, an elder retirement apartment that advertises as a place for "gracious retirement living."

The move was frustrating and difficult for Rebecca because she thought that we were giving everything away. Now the move is over, she has settled down and likes our living situation.

As Christmas comes, we rejoice in knowing that there is love all about us. That's what Christmas is all about. We pray that the Heart of Christmas will be in your home and your heart.

—Rebecca and Jo

1991: Rebecca has become a little more confused and dependent upon me for everything. She went everywhere that I went but wanted us to stay home most of the time. The children insisted that I investigate a healthcare facility. After long hours of anguished prayer, I selected one that had a personal care bed. On October 3rd, I made the hardest and saddest decision of my life—to take Rebecca to the Christian Health Center.

Within three days, the nurses said that Rebecca couldn't care for herself and that she would have to move to intermediate care. My life has changed, for we did everything together. My ministry was always a coministry.

We wish for you a Merry Christmas and may the Spirit of the Christ child be in your heart.

—Rebecca and Jo

1992: My daughter Lucinda and her son Josh took the nice "old man" on a family hiking trip and camping trip in August to the Cascade Mountains of Washington state. We hiked every day. Oh, by the way, Corky, our little dog, was given away. Now I am all alone. . . . In the spring and fall, I enrolled in a UK [University of Kentucky] class that meets twice a week. We hope for every one of you a Joyful and Peaceful Christmas.

—Rebecca and Jo

1993: As understanding and love come down at this season, it has strengthened our family relationships, and at Christmas time we pause to remember what has happened to the Riley family during 1993.

Our primary concern is Rebecca who remains at Christian Health Center. Her health is still good, but we do not take her out of the center often.

I go twice a day to feed her. While she is walking, she notices other patients in wheelchairs and tries talking to them. She doesn't recognize anyone but me and sometimes not even me.

During the year, I haven't allowed much grass to grow under my feet, attending Elder Hostels on Catalina Island, California, and at the Art Institute in Chicago.

I want all of us to feel the Spirit of Christmas and in our hearts to experience the Love, the Hope, and Faith of a Joyful Christmas.

Yours in Christmas love,

—Rebecca and Jo

1994: Christmas is all about Good News and has joy for its theme. Throughout the past year, we all have had our "ups and downs," but when we recall the message of Christmas, we can have truly a spirit of Hope.

My schedule has revolved around going to visit Rebecca. She brightens up when she sees me but hasn't called my name for more than a year and a half. (I doubt she knows me but laughs and smiles as she recognizes me as a person who comes to see her.)

In March, I spent a week in Florida as a volunteer for Habitat for Humanity. In May, a reporter from the Lexington newspaper interviewed several of us from Richmond Place who have bequeathed their brains at death to Alzheimer's research. There was a large picture of me and two others in the magazine section. I said I wasn't quite yet ready to give up my brain!

May you find the spirit of Love and a feeling of Hope this Christmas.

—*Jo*

1995: Love is what makes the world go round is a line of an old song. That's what Christmas is all about: Love—the glue that ties a family together, the bond between friends, the goodness that we express to others, the caring for others, and the spirit of friendship.

At the time of our 50th wedding anniversary all of the children surprised us with a visit. On Saturday noon we decided to have a picnic in the park as it was a beautiful day. We took Rebecca out. We hope she enjoyed it. That evening, they surprised me with a dinner with many close friends. The evening added to my special recollections of Rebecca.

Josh, our grandson, and I had a trip in October we will never forget. We traveled 1,000 miles by van to Churchill, Canada, to see polar bears in migration. We saw six polar bears and two white foxes.

At this Christmas season, I wish for you all the Christmas Joy and Love.

—*Jo*

1996: The Christmas message is a time for growing. Most of nature is dormant at this season of the year but Christmas captures our imagination and fills us with hope. Virginia Bell and David Troxel have written a book this year, *The Best Friends Approach to Alzheimer's Care*. Rebecca's life will live on in this book.

You will note that I keep busy for an old man. Besides the computer course, I attend the Donavan Forum at the University of Kentucky twice a week, and I spend as much time with the children as possible.

I hope for you the love of Christmas.

—*Jo*

1997: The spirit of Christmas is expressed in the words that we use in this season of joy. "Peace on Earth" is the message we sing with great expectation. I am grateful for the staff at the Christian Health Center. They are so good to Rebecca. They always have a smile for her, call her by name, often talk with her about being a nurse and give her a gentle massage, something she has done so many times for others. Rebecca had expressed early in her diagnosis her fear of not being treated as a "real person." Her caregivers work hard to make her feel special.

This Christmas all three children and their families are getting together at our son's house, and I will join them. It is difficult to think of celebrating Christmas without Rebecca being present.

May you have the spirit of Christmas, which is Peace, the gladness of Christmas, which is Hope, and the heart of Christmas, which is Love.

—*Jo*

1998: I have a list of folks I know, all written in a book. Every year at Christmastime I take a look and that is when I realize that these names are all a part, not of the book they're written in, but a part of us.

Rebecca is now confined to a wheelchair and her bed. No longer can she stand alone, and it takes two nurses to get her up, which is done three times a day. She had always been known as the "walker" at the center. I still go twice a day to be with Rebecca and feed her.

I have attended two elder hostels this year and visited with all the children. As we celebrate Christmas, may I wish for you a "Glorious Christmas."

—*Jo*

1999: The most unforgettable moment for me in 1999 was the passing of Rebecca on August 26. I stood at her bedside and saw her breathe her last breath as she slipped into eternity. What can I say about Rebecca's life? She had her faith and the lasting beauty of a gentle spirit. She demonstrated her hope through her children. She let each one develop as they wished. She practiced her love toward all people and I felt it the most.

A part of a prayer written by Rebecca included, "Father of us all take from us anxiety for tomorrow's food, clothing, and tomorrow's fate. Dissipate our preoccupation with things. We know that we will have wisdom and strength to act after we have accepted your peace."

The children and I have been overwhelmed by the expressions of sympathy that so many of you have shown to us.

Yours in Christmas love.

—*Jo*

12

TRANSFORMATIONS

Persons with Alzheimer's disease and other dementia often experience feelings of loss, isolation and loneliness, sadness, confusion, worry and anxiety, frustration, fear, paranoia, anger, and embarrassment. They can become easily overwhelmed by these feelings. And then what happens next? The answer to that question is all too familiar to many readers of this book: behaviors that are challenging for care partners to respond to, including anger and agitation or struggles with personal care, and a feeling of frustration and failure for the care partner.

When you learn and practice the Best Friends approach, you begin to learn how to provide care with "knack," that art of doing difficult things with ease. With empathy, strategic use of the Life Story, good communication, and other techniques described in this book, you can turn failure into success. Enormous challenges will continue to exist or emerge, but the Best Friends approach almost always makes things better.

One of Rebecca Riley's greatest fears was that others would not treat her as a "real person." Following are examples of how the Best Friends approach reinforced positive emotions and helped Rebecca feel valued, part of her family, and connected to the world around her. Your goal as a Best Friend is to find the ways that will produce these results in the person in your life. Then you, too, will understand how the Best Friends approach has helped Rebecca and so many others live a dignified life.

THE BEST FRIENDS APPROACH CAN TURN FEELINGS OF WORRY AND ANXIETY INTO FEELINGS OF CONTENTMENT

- Rebecca found listening to music and playing still-familiar songs on the piano soothing.
- Rebecca marveled at the beautiful sunsets at Crystal Lake.
- Rebecca delighted in simple activities such as watching birds and butterflies.
- Rebecca felt comforted when read aloud to.

THE BEST FRIENDS APPROACH CAN TURN FEELINGS OF FRUSTRATION INTO FEELINGS OF SERENITY AND PEACEFULNESS

- Rebecca loved knitting in front of a fireplace.
- Rebecca felt calm socializing in small groups instead of big parties.
- Rebecca found long walks peaceful.
- Rebecca enjoyed working in the yard at a slow pace.

THE BEST FRIENDS APPROACH CAN TURN FEELINGS OF CONFUSION INTO FEELINGS OF ORIENTATION

- Rebecca enjoyed old hobbies such as swimming, hiking, and boating when surrounded by family and friends.
- Rebecca responded well when others slowed down in conversations.
- Rebecca appreciated when day center staff gave her cues to relive important life events.
- Rebecca felt the most oriented in her long-term care community when surrounded by familiar family mementos.

THE BEST FRIENDS APPROACH CAN TURN FEELINGS OF LOSS INTO FEELINGS OF FULFILLMENT

- Rebecca gained a sense of worth from teaching a class for young adults at church for the first year after her diagnosis.
- Rebecca was pleased when her children thanked her for being such a great mom.
- Rebecca was proud of maintaining her family role as grandmother to her grandchildren.
- Rebecca felt rewarded when helping others, especially at the day center.

THE BEST FRIENDS APPROACH CAN TURN FEELINGS OF SADNESS INTO FEELINGS OF CHEERFULNESS

- Rebecca could be a "free spirit," having fun at the Crystal Lake cabin.
- Rebecca reminisced gleefully when her younger sister recalled funny childhood stories.
- Rebecca smiled when friends talked with her about her nursing career and her family, discussing the children by name.
- Rebecca felt cheered up when Jo teased about the time she tried to hike in the Grand Canyon with a cast on her leg.

THE BEST FRIENDS APPROACH CAN TURN FEELINGS OF EMBARRASSMENT INTO FEELINGS OF CONFIDENCE

- Rebecca liked it when Jo helped her prepare simple meals.
- Rebecca did not get embarrassed by small gaffes because her friends were so understanding.
- Rebecca felt competent and useful when exposed to day center programs that matched her remaining skills.
- Rebecca felt more equal when Jo told a joke at his own expense.

THE BEST FRIENDS APPROACH CAN TURN FEELINGS OF PARANOIA INTO FEELINGS OF TRUST

- Rebecca felt more involved in family finances when Jo had her sign the checks he filled out to pay bills.
- Rebecca liked that Jo used "we" instead of "I" when talking about their family.
- Rebecca appreciated making decisions, even simple ones, or being asked her opinion.
- Rebecca felt that friends were *their* friends, instead of Jo's friends, when Jo asked her to contribute to the annual Christmas letter.

THE BEST FRIENDS APPROACH CAN TURN FEELINGS OF FEAR INTO FEELINGS OF SECURITY

- Rebecca felt more secure when friends and families acknowledged her illness.
- Rebecca appreciated that she was never left alone in public.
- Rebecca felt reassured by friendly hugs.
- Rebecca loved feeling "protected" by her dog, Corky.

THE BEST FRIENDS APPROACH CAN TURN FEELINGS OF ANGER INTO FEELINGS OF CALM

- Rebecca released pent-up energy when walking the dog.
- Rebecca felt adequate when volunteers at the day center let her hang up her own coat.
- Rebecca found that vigorous exercise diffused anger.
- Rebecca felt distracted from her agitation by the simple act of holding hands, cuddling, or being loved.

THE BEST FRIENDS APPROACH CAN TURN FEELINGS OF ISOLATION AND LONELINESS INTO FEELINGS OF CONNECTEDNESS

- Rebecca felt important and competent when Jo made her feel part of his ministry.
- Rebecca felt friendship and support from a couples group.
- Rebecca received unconditional love from her dog, Corky.
- Rebecca felt heard when friends let her talk about the experience of Alzheimer's.
- Rebecca felt connected to God when she worshipped in her church.

The Best Friends approach transformed Rebecca by helping her operate at her best, despite her younger-onset Alzheimer's disease diagnosis. Good communication, social engagement, and friendship helped her to be happy and feel safe, secure, and valued.

The Best Friends approach also transformed her husband, Jo, helping him overcome the despair that can overwhelm families and allowing him to be his own Best Friend. According to his holiday letters during his wife's journey with Alzheimer's, Jo still managed to spend time with Rebecca at their cabin at Crystal Lake, be active in his church, enroll in a class, travel (after she moved to assisted living), spend time with family, and have some fun. He did this while still being fully engaged as Rebecca's care partner.

Think of the Best Friends approach as a road map. It is not only a way to get the person from "here" to "there," but it is also a way to bring all those who provide care from "here" to "there." This approach can shift negative behavior to positive behavior for everyone. It makes the journey of the disease more of a shared experience between the person and his or her care partner.

Family and professional care partners with knack are confident people who deliver confident care, prevent problems before they occur, and enjoy spending time with the person in their care. When care partners are not well informed, argue and correct the person with dementia, do not utilize resources, and do not take care of themselves, the darkness and despair that can come with dementia will win out.

As we conclude, we want to introduce you to one last family member who has embraced the transformative power of the Best Friends approach:

Howard Woods amazed his friends and family with his daily care of his wife, Emma, who had late-stage Alzheimer's disease. He told friends that they had not really had the best marriage, often having disagreements. Yet he said that through his time with her, caring about her, and doing things for her that he could never imagine doing for anyone, he had fallen in love with her all over again.

Remember, the medical condition of Alzheimer's disease and other dementia will not change, but your approach as care partners can. By following the Best Friends approach, you will help reduce challenging behaviors and create a joyful, safe, secure, rich, and dignified life for the person and for yourself.

There is great value in being totally present for another human being. There is great value in getting the most out of every moment, every day. There is great value in good communication. There is great value in honoring an individual's Life Story. There is great value in giving care to another.

Because any of us can be touched by Alzheimer's disease or dementia and can have times of challenge and great need, the ultimate message the authors wish to convey is this: we should treat everyone important to us as a Best Friend.

RESOURCES

Strategic Use of Community Resources

Some family members providing care for persons with dementia try to go it alone. They are resistant to using services, don't have a game plan, wait and wait to use services, and then are typically forced to make decisions around services in a crisis.

Successful care partners are strategic in their use of community-based services and programs. They undertake research to identify programs, they make a game plan, and they start to get help early in the journey.

This benefits the person with dementia and it gives friends and family needed respite.

Here are some of the most common services and programs that can help.

Adult Day Services

As mentioned in Chapter 10, we are strong advocates of adult day services, which we consider a "treatment" for dementia. Adult day centers provide supervision and enrichment for older people while giving care partners a break. Center staff can also help families link up with other community services. Some centers are dementia-specific, whereas others combine frail older people and people with cognitive losses. Readers who have a day center in their area should pay a visit today. See more at www.nadsa.org.

Alzheimer's Association Trial Match™

TrialMatch™ is a free service that makes it easy to locate clinical trials based on personal criteria and location. By participating in a clinical trial, you can help move research forward. See www.alz.org/trialmatch.

Area Agencies on Aging (AAA)

Area Agencies on Aging (AAA) are the conduits for federal, state, and local funds for community programs for older adults. AAA's also advocate for improved services for older adults and most offer a comprehensive array of services, including legal services, insurance counseling, information and referral services, and care management programs. The AAA for your region can provide you with needed assistance or refer you to reputable local providers. See more at www.n4a.org/answers-on-aging.

Church and Interfaith Volunteer Programs

Many churches have responded to the aging of the American population with services specifically aimed at older adults. For example, the number of parish nurses has increased. Also, churches sometimes use volunteers who travel to a caregiver's home to provide respite. Readers who are members of a faith community can use this community for support.

Elder Abuse Intervention Services/ Adult Protective Services

Elder abuse intervention programs investigate charges of elder mistreatment, including violence or neglect. These programs also investigate financial abuse or exploitation, a growing problem. Another name for this service is Adult Protective Services (APS); most APS programs are part of a local government and have ties to law enforcement.

See more about this important service at www.apsnetwork.org/national_resources/aps_resource_center.htm.

Friendly Visiting

Some government and private organizations have friendly visiting programs in which paid workers or volunteers make regular visits to a homebound person to spend time with him or her and make certain all is well. Some programs offer a Senior Peer Counseling program, through which trained volunteers offer support and guidance (see Senior Peer Counseling below). Check with your local Alzheimer's Association or AAA for services in your area.

Geriatric Assessment Programs/Nurses

Some private and government agencies employ individuals or teams that make home visits to assess the health of an older adult and make recommendations for needed services. There may be a charge for the assessment. These same groups may also have psychiatric assessment personnel or teams that can help evaluate if people are a danger to themselves or others.

Geriatric Care Managers

Geriatric care managers are individuals who will help set up services, handle bill paying, and provide care advice for an hourly fee. The typical care manager is a registered nurse or social worker. Caregivers should select companies or individuals who are members of the National Association of Professional Geriatric Care Managers and check references. Geriatric care management can be particularly valuable for long-distance caregivers who want a responsible party to be able to "look in on Mom (or Dad)" or for working caregivers who can afford to pay someone to help develop a care plan. These managers can also help with hiring in-home help and with residential care community placement.

See more at www.caremanager.org.

Hospice Care

Hospice programs provide dignified end-of-life care for people with dementia and support for friends and family. Hospice workers are funded by insurance or Medicare to provide medical and social support for individuals who are terminally ill and for their caregivers. Much of their focus is on providing both physical and emotional comfort. Hospice programs also have bereavement groups that can be helpful after a loved one has died.

In-Home Workers and Services

In-home staffing companies (sometimes called homemaker services) hire, train, and supervise workers who go into the home to help older adults with household chores such as laundry, shopping, cooking, and cleaning. They can also be hired to take care of personal tasks such as bathing, dressing, hair care, eating, and other personal care activities. These workers may also drive their clients to appointments or social functions. Many companies have now developed specific dementia care training for their staff; this training helps staff members understand and manage behaviors that are challenging and also teaches them the importance of socialization and activity.

Most of these companies offer nonmedical support, but some also offer nursing support to help with some medical needs of clients, such as medication management, diabetes control, and other issues. For more about these programs, see Visiting Nurse Associations (below).

Nutritional Programs and Home-Delivered Meals

Many communities have "nutrition sites" where older adults can go for a free or low-cost meal. Meals on Wheels is a well-known food delivery service that may be available in your area for adults who are homebound.

Overnight, Weekend, or Short-Term Respite Care Programs

Some residential care communities offer overnight, weekend, or short-term care. This can be invaluable if you need some time away for a family visit, have an emergency, or just need to take a vacation.

Medic Alert™ + Safe Return

Medic Alert™+ Safe Return is a program supported by the National Alzheimer's Association to help locate individuals with dementia who have wandered. This program includes a helpful kit of iron-on clothing labels and an identification bracelet. It can be an important service if you are caring for someone who wanders. Contact your local Alzheimer's Association or the National Alzheimer's Association headquarters for more information. More information can be found at www.alz.org/safetycenter.

Senior Centers

Senior centers are often the focal point in a community for older adult services and activities. At a senior center, for example, a family might find a helpful booklet on how to hire in-home help. Families should visit the centers to learn about their programs and to see if any of the activities might be appropriate for the person.

Senior Peer Counseling

Some communities have developed peer counseling programs that can send a trained volunteer to an individual's home to offer guidance and counseling. The "peer" counselor is usually a trained volunteer who is often a senior citizen or someone who has gone through a similar caregiving experience. Many family members find counseling services an invaluable way of coping with the changes in their lives, grief issues, and family conflict.

University-Based Memory Disorder Clinics

Many universities have developed specialized memory disorder clinics as part of an overall research effort. These clinics often have a team approach to care, with physicians, nurses, social workers, and neuropsychologists operating as part of a coordinated effort to make a diagnosis and provide continuing support to families. The clinics also take part in experimental drug and other research studies.

Find your nearest university center at www.alzheimers.org.

Veterans' Administration (VA) Programs

Veterans have a variety of benefits that can include long-term care. In recent years, the VA has enhanced its programs for veterans with dementia. Even if your loved one was only in the military for a short period of time, he or she may be eligible for very valuable benefits and support. A local office may be near you; check your telephone directory. For more about the VA, see www.va.gov.

Visiting Nurse Associations/ Home Health Agencies

Many visiting nurse associations/home health agencies (nonprofit and for-profit) can come to the person's home to assess his or her physical health or to provide ongoing services. Services are often covered by Medicare and private insurance. Many home health agencies schedule an initial visit to make an assessment of the person and to open a case file. Having this case file can be a lifesaver in an emergency, such as a caregiver's illness. The agency can then initiate services and will already have family contact numbers, doctors' names, and medical information.

ORGANIZATIONS, WEBSITES, AND RECOMMENDED READINGS

ORGANIZATIONS

Alzheimer's Association
225 N. Michigan Ave., Fl. 17, Chicago, IL 60601
1 800-272-3900 or 312-335-8700
www.alz.org

The national network of chapters of the Alzheimer's Association should be the first resource families turn to for help. Association chapters provide unbiased information and referrals. They offer many services in the areas of education, patient and family services, advocacy, and support for research. Their chapter-sponsored support groups, newsletters, Medic Alert™ + Safe Return program, and national 24-hour telephone Help-Line (with well-trained staff members) are particularly helpful.

Classes sponsored by the Association may change over time but recent offerings included:

Know the 10 Signs: Early Detection Matters

A class about the warning signs of Alzheimer's disease.

Understanding Memory Loss, Alzheimer's Disease and Dementia: The Basics

This program provides information on detection, causes, risk factors, stages and treatment of Alzheimer's disease.

Living with Alzheimer's Disease for People with Alzheimer's

A three-part class for persons with Alzheimer's disease.

Living with Alzheimer's for Caregivers

A series of education programs that provide answers to the questions that arise in the early, middle, and late stages of the disease. Hear from those directly affected and learn what you need to know, what you need to plan, and what you can do at each point along the way.

Legal and Financial Planning for Alzheimer's Disease

A class covering legal and financial basics.

Alzheimer's Disease Education & Referral (ADEAR) Center

www.alzheimers.org

Funded by the U.S. government's National Institute on Aging (NIA), ADEAR maintains information on Alzheimer's disease research, diagnosis, treatment, drugs, clinical trials, and federal government programs and resources. ADEAR can also help you find your nearest Alzheimer's Disease Research Center funded by NIA, most of which have memory disorder clinics.

Alzheimer's Foundation of America

www.alzfdn.org

AFA unites more than 1,600 member organizations from coast to coast that are dedicated to meeting the educational, social, emotional, and practical needs of individuals with Alzheimer's disease and related illnesses, and of their caregivers and families. Particularly helpful are links to Alzheimer's societies, day centers, and care management organizations, often in more rural areas.

AARP

www.aarp.org

http://www.aarp.org/health/brain-health/

AARP offers an excellent website with lots of information about aging and senior services. Particularly interesting is the section devoted to healthy brains.

Eldercare Locator
www.eldercare.gov
1.800.677.1116

This toll-free number and website help people locate aging services in every community throughout the United States. It is funded by the U.S. Administration on Aging. The database also includes special-purpose information and referral telephone numbers for Alzheimer's hotlines, adult day care and respite services, nursing home ombudsman assistance, consumer fraud, in-home care complaints, legal services, elder abuse/protective services, Medicare/Medicaid/Medigap information, tax assistance, and transportation. The Eldercare Locator is available weekdays, 9:00 AM to 8:00 PM (ET).

Family Caregiver Alliance
www.caregiver.org

A well-regarded national, nonprofit organization that helps caregivers coping with a variety of issues. Useful information for gay and lesbian caregivers is also on the site.

U.S. Department of Health and Human Services
www.alzheimers.gov

This website, managed by the U.S. Department of Health and Human Services, offers free information and resources about Alzheimer's disease. Here you can find links to authoritative, up-to-date information from agencies and organizations with expertise in all areas of Alzheimer's disease.

ADDITIONAL WEBSITES/WEB RESOURCES

The World Wide Web provides an amazing array of resources with information about all aspects of Alzheimer's disease and dementia. Be sure to seek out only reputable sources, however. Here are some recommended websites.

www.bestfriendsapproach.com

The official website for Virginia Bell and David Troxel's Best Friends approach includes the basics about their philosophy of care, free-of-charge downloads, information about books and publications, updates on new resources and publications, and contact information for the authors. The authors also have a Facebook "Fan Page" that can be accessed at www.facebook.com/bestfriendsapproach.

www.alz.co.uk

The Alzheimer's Disease International (ADI) site links to more than 75 Alzheimer's disease associations throughout the world. The website is rich in newsletters, publications, and helpful advice.

www.benefitscheckup.org

Benefits Checkup, a program of the National Council on Aging and other partners, is a free, easy-to-use service that identifies federal and state assistance programs for older Americans. Researching these programs used to be a time-consuming, frustrating experience; this site makes it easier.

www.dasninternational.org

Resources and networking for persons with dementia, run by persons with dementia.

www.mayoclinic.com

The well-regarded Mayo Clinic's website is another excellent resource with user-friendly articles on various aspects of dementia research, diagnosis, and treatment. Mayo Clinic's e-newsletter is available free of charge through the website.

RECOMMENDED READINGS

General Reading

Barrick, A., Rader, J., Hoeffer, D., Sloane, P., and Biddle, S. (2008). *Bathing without a battle: Person-directed care of individuals with dementia,* 2nd ed. New York: Springer Publishing Company.

Bell, V., and Troxel, D. (2001). *The best friends staff: Building a culture of care in Alzheimer's programs.* Baltimore: Health Professions Press.

Bell, V., and Troxel, D. (2004). *The best friends book of Alzheimer's activities* (vol. 1). Baltimore: Health Professions Press.

Bell, V., and Troxel, D. (2008). *The best friends book of Alzheimer's activities* (vol. 2). Baltimore: Health Professions Press.

Canfield, J. (2004). *Chicken soup for the caregiver's soul: Stories to inspire caregivers in the home, the community and the world.* Deerfield Beach, FL: Health Communications, Inc.

de Geest, G. (2007). *The living dementia case-study approach: Caregivers discover what works and what doesn't.* Vancouver, BC, Canada: Trafford Publishing.

Fazio, S., Seman, D., and Stansell, J. (1999). *Rethinking Alzheimer's care.* Baltimore: Health Professions Press.

Genova, L. (2007). *Still Alice.* New York: Simon and Schuster.

Huebner, B., ed. (2012). *I remember better when I paint.* Glen Echo, MD: Bethesda Communications Group and New Publishing Partners.

Kitwood, T. (1997). *Dementia reconsidered.* Birmingham, UK: Open University Press.

Kuhn, D. (2003). *Alzheimer's early stages: First steps in caring and treatment,* 2nd ed. Alameda, CA: Hunter House.

Laurenhue, K. (2007). *Getting to know the life stories of older adults: Activities for building relationships.* Baltimore: Health Professions Press.

Lustbader, W. (2011). *Life gets better: The unexpected pleasures of growing older*. New York: Penguin Group.

Mayo Clinic. (2009). *Mayo clinic book on Alzheimer's disease*. Rochester, MN: Mayo Clinic.

Post, S. (2000). *The moral challenge of Alzheimer's disease: Ethical issues from diagnosis to dying,* 2nd ed. Baltimore: Johns Hopkins University Press.

Power, G. Allen (2010). *Dementia beyond drugs: Changing the culture of care*. Baltimore: Health Professions Press.

Robinson A., Spencer B., and White, L. (1996). *Understanding difficult behaviors*. Ypsilanti: Eastern Michigan University.

Sheehy, G. (2010). *Passages in caregiving: Turning chaos into confidence*. New York: William Morrow.

Shenk, David. (2001). *The forgetting*. New York: Doubleday.

Sifton, C. (2004). *Navigating the Alzheimer's disease journey: A compass for caregiving*. Baltimore: Health Professions Press.

Snyder, L. (2010). *Living your best with early stage Alzheimer's*. North Beach, MN: Sunrise River Press.

Thomas, W. (2004). *What are old people for? How elders will save the world.* Acton, MA: VanderWyk & Burnham.

Warner, M. L. (2000). *The complete guide to Alzheimer's-proofing your home,* revised ed. West Lafayette, IN: Purdue University Press.

White, L., and Spencer, B. (2000). *Moving a relative with memory loss: A family caregiver's guide*. Santa Rosa, CA: Whisp Publications.

Personal Accounts

Avadian, B. (2005). *Where's my shoes? My father's walk through Alzheimer's.* Lancaster, CA: North Star Books.

Debaggio, T. (2002). *Losing my mind: An intimate look at life with Alzheimer's*. New York: The Free Press.

Peterson, B. (2010). *Jan's story: Love lost to the long goodbye of Alzheimer's*. Lake Forest, CA: Behler Publications.

Snyder, L. (2009). *Speaking our minds: What it's like to have Alzheimer's*, revised ed. Baltimore: Health Professions Press.

Taylor, R. (2006). *Alzheimer's from the inside out*. Baltimore: Health Professions Press.

Just for Children

Fox, M., and Vivas. J. (1989). *Wilfrid Gordon McDonald Partridge* (Public Television Storytime Books). San Diego, CA: Kane/Miller Book Publishers.

Shriver, M., and Speidel, S. (2004). *What's happening to Grandpa?* New York: Little Brown and Company and Warner Books.

Other Resources/Tools

The Alzheimer's Store—www.alzstore.com—A wonderful resource with home safety products, books and resources, and activity ideas.

Caring Cards—a handy set of cards with ideas to start a meaningful conversation. www.dramycaregiving.com.

Scramble Squares—Easy-to-use puzzles on a variety of themes and topics.

www.b-dazzle.com. See also http://www.wisernow.com/PDF/Scramble Squaresdescription.pdf.

Wiser Now—A rich resource of booklets and activity ideas. www.wisernow.com.

BIOGRAPHIES

Claralee Arnold (1926–2005)

Music and family paint the picture of Claralee's life. She sang in the choir of Transylvania University and graduated with a degree in music. She continued her musical career by giving private piano lessons in her home. For fifty years, she sang in her church choir, always a highlight of her week. When her mother was having problems with her memory, Claralee would spend hours playing the piano and singing songs with her. They both loved music.

Her husband, Clyde, and their three sons, Stephen, David, and Richard, all Eagle Scouts, were her pride and joy. The family enjoyed bowling together, and some members were golfers. Claralee had a hole-in-one to her credit. She was fun-loving and had been a Best Friend to many. (p. 205)

Gladys Bell (1923–2005)

His Harley Davidson motorcycle was very impressive, but most of all, Gladys was in love with the owner, a young man named Kenneth Bell. After she graduated from high school, they were married by an uncle who was a Baptist minister. Gladys worked during the day and continued her education by taking classes at night.

After a brief tour in the Army, Gladys and Kenneth settled in Lexington, Kentucky. They had two children, Cathy and Bradley. For thirty-five years, Kenneth worked for a standard-bred racehorse firm. They had four grandchildren and one great-granddaughter.

Gladys always enjoyed various kinds of handwork, including sewing, knitting, needlepoint, and quilting. She made several quilts for her children and grandchildren. Gladys and Kenneth were active members of their church. Her husband described her as "getting along with everyone, because of her friendly nature." (p. 118)

Margaret Brubaker (1907–1996)

Margaret was born in Duluth, Minnesota, and moved to California at an early age. There she graduated from the famous Hollywood High. In an era when many women worked only in the home, Margaret worked in a variety of positions, including a family-owned restaurant and her father's ice cream company.

Margaret and her husband, Dudley, raised their son, James ("Jim"), in a neighborhood full of his cousins. The Brubakers lived next door to Dudley's sister and brother-in-law, Lois and Siegfried ("Sig") Haas, with whom they had a sixty-year friendship. Margaret was proud of Jim and his career as a movie producer and of her grandchildren, Marcei, Susan, and John.

Even late in her illness, Margaret remained interested and involved in the world around her. Her family remembers her as a "take-charge" person with a wonderful sense of humor. (pp. 93–94, 116–117)

Mary Burmaster (1914–2000)

"My name is pronounced 'BUR-master' not 'Bur-MASTER,'" Mary, a quiet, thoughtful person, always made clear. Famous American and English writers were no strangers to Mary because she was often the first to finish a familiar line from one of their works. When her daughter, Betsey, was a little girl, Mary taught her the poem that she learned when she was a little girl. She enjoyed sharing with us the Betsey version: "The North wind doth blow and we shall have snow. What will poor robin do then? He'll sit in the barn to keep himself warm and tuck his head under his wing. Poor 'shing' [instead of 'thing']."

Mary knew every word to the songs of the Big Band era. Nothing pleased her more than to sing throughout the day, unless it was to talk about her three children, Lee, Betsey, and Mary Anne. (pp. 85, 116)

John "Jack" R. Cooper Jr. (1933–2002)

Serving as a coxswain for four years on the Syracuse University rowing team was a special memory for Jack Cooper. He loved competing with many other college teams and especially hoped to win over Navy. After completing medical school, he served on a military transport ship. During this time, he traveled to many parts of the world. He was a surgeon in private practice.

Jack's wife and their two children enjoyed family times of golf, tennis, and skiing and once took a three-week trip out West, camping under the stars. Jack was a proud grandparent. Singing songs of the 1950s and familiar hymns, as well as dancing and playing the banjo and ukulele, showed the musical side of this physician.

"Thoughtful, gentle, and caring," are used by his wife to paint a "word picture" of Jack. (pp. 21, 119–120)

Brevard Crihfield (1916–1987)

Brevard, nicknamed "Crihf," took enormous pride in being reminded of his past as Executive Director of the Council of State Governments. Friends and family could remember him staying busy in various committee meetings or enjoying a break with a newspaper, a cup of coffee, and a cigarette. Crihf's early years were spent in Illinois, and he recalled "Ronnie" Reagan attending Eureka College in Illinois while he attended the University of Chicago. Family, his dog Ho, beautiful art books, and favorite poems were always topics of conversation. Another interest was baseball; he played second base like a pro.

Crihf was a very private person. When he enrolled in the Helping Hand Day Center, he approached most activities cautiously; yet, he was a superb dancer and would always embrace an opportunity to dance, especially to the music of Benny Goodman's orchestra. (pp. 18–19, 120–121)

Rubena S. Dean (1931–1999)

"The Yellow Rose of Texas" brought a big smile to Rubena's face as she recalled many happy memories of her childhood in Texas and her graduation from Texas University for Women in Denton. She loved her years of teaching physical education, English, and history to junior high school students.

Rubena enjoyed being part of a large extended family and maintained close relationships with her children, Lynn and Ted, and her grandchildren. Helping people was also a major part of her life. Her community benefited from her generosity; she was president of many service-related clubs, she organized church activities, and she volunteered in nursing facilities. Rubena thrived on hard work. Before the onset of her illness, she enjoyed hobbies such as bridge, piano, and needlepoint. (pp. 26, 93)

Letch Dixon (1932–)

Letch was the baby of twelve children. He loves to share the story that his parents "finally found out what was causing all those children!" Letch attended two years of high school and then attended a trade school. He later joined the Air Force and after his tour of duty he worked in a steel mill. Once he met Lenna, he had eyes for no one else and they became the parents of four children, Robin, Sharon, Amanda, and Marvin.

Letch and his family enjoy taking trips to Yellowstone, Canada, and Florida. He and his wife love music, especially bluegrass, and Letch is a clogger. He also likes to fish and hunt and has bagged four elk in Colorado. Letch is easygoing and very witty. He likes to share his funny stories about growing up in such a large family. (p. 207)

Edna Denton Edwards (1909–2003)

Edna was proud to be part of a tradition of three generations of third-grade teachers; she followed her mother, and her daughter, Peggy, followed her. Edna had many talents; she was an artist (her artwork is on the cover of *Activity Programming for Persons with Dementia: A Source Book*, published by the national Alzheimer's Association), a pianist, a seamstress, and a good cook, known for making an excellent corn pudding.

After her husband died at a relatively young age, Edna was both mother and father to their daughters, Patricia, Peggy, and Janet. The Immanuel Baptist Church was her tower of strength.

Edna was highly competitive, was a big tease, loved to clown around, and made friends easily. (p. 84)

Hobert Elam (1917–2003)

A "dyed in the wool" Kentuckian, Hobert Elam was proud to be living on his farm surrounded by his Angus cattle. He remembered spending time as a child with his grandfather, and by the time he was10 years old, he was helping his father build houses. He explained, "Life was simple then. We were excited to receive oranges and candy in our stockings at Christmas."

Hobert served as an engineer in World War II and afterward met his wife, Irene. They had two children and five grandchildren. He was a home-builder, a real estate investor, and a cattle farmer. He loved singing, especially the hymns of his faith, as well as working on the family genealogy, gardening, and being with his family. Hobert was a "people person." He could make friends with the young and the old. (p. 23)

Mary Edith Engle (1916–2003)

If Mary Edith hadn't stood on tiptoe she would never have passed the test for height to become a pilot during World War II as a member of the Woman's Air Force Service Pilots (WASPs). She ferried planes—from tiny cub fighters to B-29 bombers—from the factory to military bases all over the United States.

Her husband, three daughters, and grandchildren were central in her life. Her many other interests included gardening, music, traveling, boating, training and racing saddle-bred horses, and painting. Mary Edith was often described as "spunky," and to honor her adventuresome spirit in flying, she was inducted into the Kentucky Aviation Hall of Fame in 1997. She looked back on her life saying, "We've had a great life. . . . I don't think I'd do anything different." (pp. 76–77)

Patricia Estill (1938–2010)

Patricia was born in Kentucky and remained a staunch supporter of all that is Kentucky. She married her high school sweetheart and they became parents of two girls, Sheri and Paulette. Later her three granddaughters became the "apples of her eye." She taught school for a while and then became a dental assistant.

Patricia was born an artist and she felt most at home all her life with a paint brush. She enjoyed being an artist to the very end of her life. She was also very musical, loving to dance and sing, especially the hymns of her faith. She had a "thing" for colorful clothes and "one of a kind" earrings. Patricia loved life. She had an irresistible smile, a contagious laugh, and a hug for everyone. (p. 208)

Marydean Evans (1910–1997)

"Did you really 'pogo' down Broadway and in the front window of your father's sporting goods store?" a friend of Marydean's once asked in disbelief. Marydean's father had the latest equipment, including the first pogo stick in Kentucky. She and her four brothers and sisters helped publicize this new contraption.

Swimming, dancing (she was known as the best dancer at the famous Brown Hotel's Roof Garden in Louisville, Kentucky), and preparing fancy food as a caterer were some of Marydean's accomplishments. Chocolate in any form was a favorite food, and butter was a close second. "Bread is just a vehicle to deliver butter," she admitted with a grin.

Marydean was a cheerful person. Her children, Betty, Tip, and Ann, and her grandchildren provided strong support. They were proud of her volunteer work. (pp. 78, 92)

Henrietta Frazier (1921–2003)

"Our house has always been for everyone." Henrietta was proud that her house was home base for family and friends. The youngest of six children, she enjoyed all the comings and goings in a close extended family. With a nursing degree from St. Elizabeth's Hospital School of Nursing, Henrietta served both the private and public sectors in a caring, thoughtful, and dedicated manner.

When she was four years old, Henrietta had to have an eye removed. Despite her vision impairment, she embraced life fully. She had a jolly disposition, with a quick wit.

She and her sister, Mae, traveled extensively and especially enjoyed cruises. Because they lived together, they shared many close friends. Henrietta was an avid fan of basketball and joined many clubs and causes. (pp. 25, 103)

Sergio (Serge) Torres Gajardo (1920–1995)

Serge was always a big tease! "I left Chile because one day when I was piloting a small plane, I swooped down over a chicken coop, crashed my plane, and killed all the chickens." Serge was a second lieutenant in the Chilean Air Force before becoming an American citizen.

His family included his wife, Gertrude; their three children, Roxanne, Suzi, and John; and three grandchildren. They vacationed together in a favorite spot in Mexico and were active in all aspects of their church.

Music was woven into Serge's life in many ways. He loved to dance to the rhythms of Latin music. He enjoyed a wide range of songs, from Big Band to classical to opera. Playing tennis and Ping-Pong and following the Chicago Cubs and the Green Bay Packers gave him great pleasure. He also liked to fish, hunt, swim, and read. Serge was affectionate, unselfish, and full of fun. (pp. 80, 81)

Edna Carroll Greenwade (1916–1996)

Edna Carroll grew up on a farm, the youngest of five brothers and sisters. Edna Carroll enjoyed being teased: "Did your brothers and sisters spoil you?" She denied being spoiled, but in fact had many memories of being the "baby doll" in the family. Her daughter, Katie, grandchildren, and one great-grandson were central to her life.

Helping and caring about others were a great part of Edna Carroll's life. She was active in her church, helping to cook special dinners. A library of recipes stood ready for her to share a dish of food for any occasion. She enjoyed sewing, quilting, and working with ceramics. A loving person, Edna Carroll was anxious to please, friendly, and fun. (pp. 89–90)

Geri Greenway (1940–1997)

"That is van Gogh's *The Starry Night*," Geri might quickly point out when leafing through a beautiful book of paintings. The worlds of art, literature, and opera were familiar territory for her. Impressively, she read about those subjects in several languages.

After earning a PhD in German literature, she taught at several colleges. She endeared herself to her students with her extensive knowledge and her ability to teach her subjects in a relaxed atmosphere.

Geri was proud of her family, and together they enjoyed traveling, swimming, gardening, and jogging. Adopting a whale named Olympia was just one expression of Geri's ecological concern. She enjoyed Cajun food, a taste from her birth state of Louisiana. Talented, sophisticated, beautiful, and loving described Geri. (pp. 22, 96)

Edith Hayes (1919–2005)

"Here comes Edith, our chief hugger." And what warm, reassuring hugs she had for everyone! Edith was born on a farm near Corning, Iowa, one of nine children. Her family valued education, and Edith earned her nursing degree at the University of Missouri. She put this training to good use as the college nurse at Alice Lloyd College in Kentucky where her husband was president. Their five children would also tell you that she practiced her nursing on all of them.

Simplicity in all of life describes Edith. She delighted in birdsongs, rejoiced in the first spring flowers, was a prolific note writer and made her own cards, and loved being with her children, grandchildren, and great-grandchildren. (pp. 94, 114, 214–215)

James Holloway (1927–2002)

Being president of his fifth-grade class showed Jim Holloway's early love of school and education. Enlisting in the Army after high school graduation opened up many opportunities for him to further pursue this interest through the G.I. Bill. He attended Howard and Vanderbilt Universities and later received his PhD from Yale University. While at Yale, he met his wife to be, Nancy. They were the parents of three children.

Jim taught philosophy and religion at the university level. He was a biblical scholar, loving to spend hours discussing the views of the great religious writers through the ages. He spent a year in Basel, Switzerland, studying theology under Karl Barth, one of the great theologians of the twentieth century. He cherished keeping up with some of his friends from his days at Yale, as well as traveling and visiting art museums. (pp. 86, 203)

Frances (Annie) Holman (1933–2002)

Summer on the farm with her grandparents was a fun time for Annie, a city girl. She loved riding her bicycle in the wide-open spaces. After graduating from high school, she attended a four-year nursing program and became a surgical nurse.

It was love at first sight on a blind date, and Annie and Jack Holman were married within the year. They had three daughters and four grandchildren. They both enjoyed traveling, bowling, and dancing—from line dancing and clogging to ballroom. Their church and their family were central in their lives. Annie endeared herself to those around her with her contagious smile and affectionate manner. (pp. 25, 213)

Dicy Bell Reed Jenkins (1902–1991)

Born in the Oklahoma Territory before Oklahoma became a state, Dicy liked to recall her early childhood living in tents and covered wagons. She bragged that she could do everything her eight brothers did, including chopping and hauling wood and working in the fields.

Dicy amazed everyone with her catalog of old sayings. When asked how she was feeling, she always said, "A little better than a blank." Other expressions that she used often were “No fool, no fun,” “mother wit,” and “there’s no fool like an old fool.” Feisty at times, shaking her cane to make a point, Dicy endeared herself to everyone. Dicy and her husband, Lawrence, had two children, Lawrencetta and Edward, and raised two granddaughters, Nawanta and Nelvean. Dicy lived with Nawanta during the last years of her life. A devoted family and a strong faith in God sustained Dicy through good and bad times. (pp. 95, 250)

Leota Kilkenny (1903–1994)

“St. John, Kentucky. That’s close to Louisville.” Leota enjoyed recalling her early years on the farm near St. John. The boys milked the cows, and the milk was shipped by train to Louisville. She had vivid memories of being invited to ride to the station and watch as the milk was loaded on the train. She loved the farm, especially the animals and the woods near the house, where she played with many brothers and sisters. Leota graduated from high school at nearby Bethlehem Academy.

A full-time homemaker, Leota was a dedicated wife and mother of three children: Ann Marie, John, and Mary Jane. She and her family were active in the Roman Catholic Church. Always ready to give a hug, she was kind, thoughtful, and fun-loving. (pp. 77–78)

John Lackey, (1944–)

John is the only child of an only child of an only child. He enjoys talking about how special it has always been to have so much attention. It was love at first sight when he met his wife to be, Sherry, while still in high school. They married at a very early age and became the parents of three children—Jeff, John, and Jennifer. He majored in education in college and became a teacher for the rest of his working life. In 2006 John retired after teaching for forty years. While teaching he did some coaching in football and basketball, and even coached the school chess club.

John loves working on his family’s genealogy and an occasional trip to Las Vegas. John is an artist at heart. He sees joy in the miracles of nature and loves nothing better than a beautiful sunset, often calling the family to a "sunset alert." He is also an artist at being a kind, gentle, and loving friend. (p. 209)

Masanori (Mas) Matsumura (1937–2008)

Born in Santa Monica, California, "Mas" Matsumura was the oldest of three children and part of a close-knit family. He was five years old when his family was interned in Manzanar, California, during World War II. Notably, the photographer Ansel Adams took his portrait during that time. As a young man, Mas was very athletic and motivated.

He was married to his wife, May, for over forty years. They had three children, Cindy, Donna, and Riki. Before retiring in 1993, Mas worked in a commercial nursery business that specializes in gardenias.

His children say that Mas was always there for them. "A friendly and gentle spirit" is a description that comes to mind whenever one thinks of Mas. (pp. 79, 91–92)

Willa Lee McCabe (1915–1997)

"Sometimes the little ones cried on the first day of school. I just hugged and hugged them." Willa, a first-grade teacher for thirty-two years, knew exactly what to do. Children, including her grandsons, Greg and Jason, were the light of Willa's life.

Willa enjoyed talking about the past, including the fun she had walking to school with her friends, taking her school lunch in a straw lunch basket, and playing games at recess. She also enjoyed talking about her special hobbies, including raising a vegetable garden and making quilts, listening to music, singing, and taking long walks. Willa's face showed a contagious burst of joy when greeting friends. She lit up the room, energizing the people around her. (p. 103)

Ruby Mae Morris (1912–1999)

A life of hard work did not dampen Ruby Mae's love of having a good time. She was a prankster and always loved a good joke. Her love of children and animals was evident: "God gave them to us to love and care for," she reminded us often. Her family, her church, and caring for others were central to her life. Ruby Mae insisted that she did not mind hard work: "Just get the paint, and I'll paint your house all the way to the roof. I can do lots of things that you don't know about." She loved to sing and dance and stayed dressed in her best clothes, "camera-ready," for her picture to be taken.

Her daughter, Dolores, praised her: "She's a very special rose in our garden, and God will pick her for an eternal garden." She had a sweet, sweet spirit. (pp. 19, 88)

Harry Nelson (1946–2012)

Harry was born in New Orleans, Louisiana, and liked to celebrate his Cajun upbringing by enjoying spicy food, music, and having fun. He attended Loyola University where he met his wife, Joan, the love of his life. After spending time in the Army, he practiced dentistry. He loved telling about making their wedding bands himself, a skill learned from his work as a dentist.

Harry was a family man and adored their two children and a grandson. He always loved the outdoors, hiking in the parks across the United States, kayaking, and gardening. Harry was a lover of music and a great dancer. He enjoyed nothing more than finding a good dance partner and losing himself in the rhythm of the music. He was a very witty and super social person. (pp. 17–18)

Jerome (Jerry) Ruttenberg (1908–1987)

A series of small strokes could not steal all of Jerry's sense of humor and amazing intellect. He had a pun for almost every occasion, and his quick wit brought joy to all. Once, when he heard the song "Cruising Down the River" being sung off-key, Jerry was quick to say, "Lifeboats, please, we're sinking." In answer to the question "What do you remember about being twelve years old?" he quipped, "Waiting to be thirteen."

He named his favorite dog Sooner, telling all that he chose this name because the dog would "rather eat sooner than later." Dancing, singing, card games, and word puzzles were relaxing to him. Jerry was an outstanding businessman, a humanitarian, an avid reader, and most of all, a devoted husband and father. (p. 91)

Maria Scorsone (1922–2005)

Born in Balestrate, Sicily, Maria had vivid memories of a childhood view—she could look out the bedroom window of their beach house and see the ocean. Music had always been a very important part of Maria's life. She had piano lessons as a child and became an accomplished pianist, a skill she enjoyed all of her life. She also enjoyed horseback riding with her father during her growing-up years.

Maria and her family lived in Argentina for many years. When the family moved to the United States, Maria finished her PhD at Syracuse University and taught Spanish and Italian at the University of Kentucky and Eastern Kentucky University. Beautiful, regal, caring, and devoted to her family described Maria. (pp. 83–84)

Emma Simpson (1921–2003)

Emma was one of the younger daughters in a family of sixteen children. She was born and raised in rural Russell County, Kentucky. She had to quit school at sixteen to go to work to help support her family. At nineteen years of age she married Leslie Simpson and eventually had two children, a girl and a boy.

Emma had always been known for her wit and sparkling personality. She regretted her lack of education and earned her GED when she was in her fifties. In addition to working for the state government, Emma found time to do volunteer work in the community. After her retirement, she and her husband spent much time at the Senior Citizens' Center in Frankfort, Kentucky, organizing dances, potluck dinners, and exercise classes, and teaching reading in an adult literacy program. (pp. 24, 89)

Robert Steele (1936–)

Robert (Bob) Steele was born in the Philippines where his father, a colonel in the U.S. Army, was stationed at the time. Bob spent much of his early life with his aunt and grandmother. After high school he enrolled at UCLA. Much to his father's disgust, he flunked out and was faced with an ultimatum to either go to work or join the military. Bob likes to tell this story. He enrolled in the Naval Academy and served with honors in the U.S. Navy.

He enjoys talking about all the places he visited while in service. He and his wife, Darlene, love to travel. A twelve-day cruise on the Rhone River is one of their favorite trips. Bob also likes Civil War history and all kinds of sports. He is easygoing and likes kidding around. (pp. 80–81)

Tap Steven (1923–)

Tap was born of missionary parents in a small medical station on a mountainside in China. He left China at age three, but never lost his passion and interest in world affairs. He later earned a PhD in International Education at the University of Southern California and devoted much of his working life to international dispute resolution, including thirteen years working with the Saudi Arabian government.

Within two years of retiring to Santa Barbara in 1996, Tap and his wife, Frankie, began noticing his lapses in memory. They have both faced his diagnosis with Alzheimer's disease head on, continuing to stay active in their retirement community, Vista del Monte. Tap also teaches for the local Adult Education program and continues writing poetry. He says, "It's important not to withdraw into the secret corners of our life, but to risk making mistakes and to keep on reaching out to friends—to partake in a full life." (pp. 82, 211)

Evelyn Merrell Talbott (1913–1992)

Evelyn was known as a bookworm even as a little girl; as she grew up, her books were her best friends. She turned this love of books into a degree in library science from the University of Kentucky. She enjoyed working as a librarian for many years. At the day center she would often announce, "I brought a new book for us to enjoy today." Soon she would be immersed in a book, such as *The Wonders of the Underwater World.*

Evelyn's dog, Willie, was very much a part of her family, which included her husband, Bob, and their daughter, Susan. Willie even traveled with the family on their favorite trip to the beach. Evelyn loved music and dancing. She was always friendly and appreciative. (pp. 84, 117)

Frances Tatman (1935–2007)

Frances's husband, William, admits that when he got to know her at activities at their church, "She caught my eye." They were married in 1953 and had four children—Laura, Amy, Theodore, and Michael—and seven grandchildren.

Frances always enjoyed the simple things in life. As a teenager, Frances delighted in being invited to visit her grandparents who lived on farms. She and her family traveled to various state parks for family picnics. Her church was an important part of her life, and the choir benefited from her beautiful voice. Frances could whistle in tune with any song and amazed her friends with her clear, bell-like solos. Frances's husband described her as being "much a lady" and a good wife and mother. (p. 96, 97)

Dorothy Troxel (1923–2008)

Dorothy Troxel was born in Vancouver, Canada, but lived much of her young life in Hong Kong. Her family lived a privileged life there until everything changed after the city fell to the Japanese in World War II. Along with the rest of the British colony, the family was interned during the war but survived to start over in Montreal. Dorothy married her husband, Fred, a career Air Force officer, and enjoyed a wonderful fifty-year-plus marriage that took the two of them all over the world.

Dorothy was an elegant, always well-dressed lady who spoke several languages and had many friends. She loved hosting a fancy tea party, sipping her favorite Earl Grey tea. She was very proud of her son, David, and his career supporting persons with dementia. (pp. 100, 210, 250)

Emma Parido Woods (1921–1992)

Emma grew up with three brothers who took good care of her when she was a little girl. After high school, she worked in the tobacco industry in the "re-drier" (where tobacco was processed for shipping) and as a timekeeper. That was hard work—Emma could attest to that!

On June 4, 1950, Emma married Howard Woods. Together they raised eight children. The parental terms of endearment given to them by the children were Big Momma and Big Daddy. Emma became a full-time homemaker, and their house became the gathering place for all, including grandchildren and great-grandchildren. Emma was devoted to her family. She also maintained a strong religious faith, enjoying listening to and singing hymns. (p. 276)

Nancy Zechman (1928–1992)

A very athletic person during her youth, Nancy chose to major in physical education at Miami University in Oxford, Ohio. Her athletic interest and ability continued throughout her life, and she had a special skill and flair for tennis.

Nancy was also an artistic person, creating a beautiful home for her husband, Fred, children, Rick and Jami, and her cats, Marilyn and Monroe. She volunteered on a regular basis at a local hospital and pursued many other interests, including attending art classes and workshops, gardening, playing cards, doing needlework, and playing sports of all varieties. Nancy's infectious smile and love of people kept her surrounded with "friends aplenty." (pp. 121, 123)

Phil Zwicke (1949–2007)

Phil Zwicke displayed an early talent for engineering when he took apart a faucet at age three. He went on to earn a BA, MA, and PhD in electrical engineering and enjoyed a successful career that included many patents and awards. He married Karen in 1991 and was dedicated to her and his two sons. After his diagnosis of Alzheimer's disease at age 49, he continued to enjoy his passions for windsurfing, long hikes with his dog, travel, and, above all, time spent with family. Phil and Karen also renewed their wedding vows, traveled to Hawaii, spent a month in Europe, and visited places they had never been, including Las Vegas and Yellowstone. Phil remained a gentle soul and was a popular member of his early-stage dementia support group. (pp. 82–83, 212)

ABOUT THE AUTHORS

Virginia Bell, MSW, has spent a lifetime being a friend to humanity. Married to a minister, she nurtured and contributed generously to her community while raising their five children. Before her husband retired, Ms. Bell pursued a master's degree in social work, which she completed in 1982 at age sixty from the University of Kentucky. She counseled families at the University of Kentucky's Sanders-Brown Center on Aging and learned to appreciate the unique challenges faced by people with Alzheimer's disease and other dementia and their care partners. Her response was to establish the Helping Hand Adult Day Center (now the Best Friends Adult Day Center) in Lexington, Kentucky, to provide the kind of care she believed these families needed most. Ms. Bell has subsequently trained innumerable staff, students, and volunteers nationally and internationally in the practices and attitudes that embody the Best Friends approach.

She has earned awards for leadership in her community and in the Alzheimer's field and has published four other books with her coauthor, David Troxel, about using the Best Friends approach in professional care settings (*The Best Friends Approach to Alzheimer's Care; The Best Friends Staff: Building a Culture of Care in Alzheimer's Programs;* and *The Best Friends Book of Alzheimer's Activities, Volumes 1 and 2;* all published by Health Professions Press).

Today, when she isn't spending time with her family, which now includes twelve grandchildren and five great-grandchildren, she is traveling around the nation and throughout the world bearing the good news that much can be done to improve the lives of those affected by Alzheimer's disease and other dementia.

With a long history in the field of public health, **David Troxel, MPH,** has dedicated his professional life to improving the well-being of the public at large and people with Alzheimer's disease and other dementia specifically. After earning his master's degree in public health, Mr. Troxel worked at the University of Kentucky Sanders-Brown Center on Aging, which at the time was one of only ten federally funded Alzheimer's research centers in the country. It was there he met and began to collaborate with Virginia Bell to improve education and services in the state of Kentucky for people with dementia and their care partners. He was the first executive director of the Lexington/Bluegrass chapter of the Alzheimer's Association (now called the Greater Kentucky and Southern Indiana chapter) and, together with Ms. Bell, he won an unprecedented four Excellence in Program Awards from the national Alzheimer's Association for his chapter's patient and family programs.

From 1994 to 2004, Mr. Troxel was Executive Director of the California Central Coast chapter (formerly the Santa Barbara & Ventura County chapters) of the Alzheimer's Association, where he developed innovative dementia care programs with a dedicated staff and group of volunteers. Today he works as a writer, speaker, and long-term care/dementia care consultant based in Sacramento, California.

Mr. Troxel has also been a family caregiver, supporting his mother, Dorothy, who passed away from Alzheimer's disease in 2008 after a ten-year journey with the disease.

In addition to the books he has co-written with Ms. Bell on their Best Friends philosophy, together they have written a series of influential journal articles on topics ranging from spirituality, to staff training and development, to person-centered care, including the widely reprinted Alzheimer's Disease Bill of Rights. A well-traveled speaker and advocate, Mr. Troxel has inspired professionals around the world to start making sorely needed changes in the culture of care for the millions of people living with dementia.

To learn more about Virginia's and David's work, visit them on the Web at www.bestfriendsapproach.com or at www.facebook.com/bestfriendsapproach.

INDEX